Girl, Wasted

A Personal Story of Addiction, Obsession, and Redemption

BRITTANY TALTOS

GIRL, WASTED: A PERSONAL STORY OF ADDICTION, OBSESSION, AND REDEMPTION
Copyright © 2020 by Brittany Taltos

All rights reserved. Printed in the United States of America. No part of this book may be used or reproduced in any manner whatsoever without written permission except in the case of brief quotations embodied in critical articles or reviews.

For more information visit: https://girlwasted.com/

Cover design by Cristian Guamanzara

ISBN: 978-0-578-72299-3

First Edition: July 2020

Table of Contents

Author's Note iii
Acknowledgements iii
Chapter 1: Rock Bottoms Up 1
Chapter 2: Cigar Smoke and Mirrors 11
Chapter 3: Shrek Is Not for Kids 27
Chapter 4: A Drunken Situation 41
Chapter 5: Bachelor Pad Blackout 57
Chapter 6: New York City of Dreams 69
Chapter 7: M Is for Men with Money 81
Chapter 8: Wet Dream Chaser 97
Chapter 9: Beauty and the Beast 103
Chapter 10: The Super Alcoholic 119
Chapter 11: The Phone Call Girl 129
Chapter 12: Dish of Dirt 137
Chapter 13: The Wife Comes to Life 147
Chapter 14: Intoxicated and Loveless 153
Chapter 15: I'm a Freaking Alcoholic 167

Chapter 16: Dry as a Bone 179

Chapter 17: Relapse Central Station 189

Chapter 18: Blood, Sweat, and Rehab 199

Chapter 19: Riding in the Druggy Buggy 209

Chapter 20: Sober-Livin' the Life 217

Chapter 21: The Secret Letter 223

Chapter 22: Love After Addiction 227

Chapter 23: Alcoholism in an Alcoholic Society 233

Chapter 24: Goodbye, Love 237

About the Author 241

Author's Note

Everything that I write about in this book actually happened, unfortunately. I am an alcoholic and alcoholics tend to black out. The events that I describe are based on my own blurry recollections.

This is *my* story.

Some names and identifying details have been changed to protect the privacy of individuals.

Acknowledgements

I dedicate this book to my mom. I apologize for any cringe-worthy material. Thank you for standing by my side every step of the way.

To the love of my life, thank you for making me a better person.

To my twin sister, thank you for loving me unconditionally.

To my brother, thank you for insipiring me.

"I understood myself only after I destroyed myself. And, in the process of fixing myself, did I know who I really was."

-Sade Andria Zabala

CHAPTER 1

Rock Bottoms Up

I opened my swollen eyes in a tiny two-bedroom apartment in Manhattan. I was sweaty and shaky and could barely use my legs to stand up. My limbs were not listening to me; no matter how hard I tried I couldn't get my dilapidated twenty-five-year-old body to do what I wanted it to do. This enraged me. I noticed my shorts were on backwards. I was surprised I was wearing any at all.

My apartment was just as disheveled as my clothing. What the hell had happened? There were empty food wrappers strewn all over, pizza crust lying beside me, and an empty bottle of vodka staring at me. That enraged me. I started cursing under my breath. I looked at my puffy, bloated hands and attempted to gauge my hangover by how many tremors I was experiencing.

I was crumbling right in front of that empty bottle of vodka. That bottle's stare haunts me to this day. It had such an absurd power over my body, mind, and soul. It dictated my every move. It distracted me from my reality and gave me a purpose to wake up in the morning.

On this morning, it was my only motivation to pull my two wobbly legs through two small pant holes. This simple task was daunting to someone who was a slave to alcohol and hadn't yet acquired their morning ritualistic dose. I needed at least one drop to function. Who am I kidding? I needed at least a healthy guzzle to muzzle my crying soul and body pangs. My body needed it to function, my mind needed it for clarity, and my soul needed it for warmth.

How does one's soul become a slave to a substance? The answer to that lies deep inside my diseased and twisted brain. I am a people pleaser. When someone would tell me to do something, I listened. As a child this was the norm. I listened to my alcoholic father to avoid chaos, and I tended to my mother to avoid guilt. I learned at an early age to tolerate those in authority. In this moment, vodka was my master.

Vodka used to whisper sweet nothings in my ear and promise me moments of carefree bliss. But this morning, it was roaring in my ear and holding my body hostage until I felt the burn of its existence in my esophagus.

I crawled to the nearest shirt. I could barely lift my arms but managed to wriggle into last night's oversized, stained men's t-shirt. It reeked of fried buffalo wings and vodka, which, in a disgusting way, motivated me to power through the suffering. When I stood, I felt the heaviness of a diseased body dominate my every move. Despite my head pounding and my inability to focus with my own two eyes, I managed to collect myself.

My face was beaded with sweat. Chunks of unwashed hair adhered to my temples. I attempted to slick all loose strands back with a flimsy hair tie. As I lifted my arms above my head, I was overcome by a wave of faintness. This seemingly simple action of securing my hair proved strenuous and painful. I breathed a sigh of relief as the weight of those strands lifted from my shoulders. I felt composed.

When I opened my foul-smelling purse, I noticed my Florida ID card still in the side pocket, untouched from the night before. A sense of pure bliss and excitement filled my decrepit body. The only thing missing was a fifty-dollar bill that I vaguely remember being there from the fuzzy night before. Sheer panic engrossed my body. Did I spend it? Did someone steal it? Or did I give it to a homeless person begging on the street last night? That question will forever be a mystery. It went into my stockpile of forgotten memories of blacked-out nights and drunken escapades.

After scrounging up quarters from the pant pockets of my roommate, I headed to the liquor store. As the elevator door swung open to an array of work-goers, my heart sank. I tried to catch the next elevator, but everybody politely insisted that I squeeze in. This terrifying moment burned into my brain. Could they smell the stench of fermented vodka on my stained shirt? Could they sniff my alcoholism through their thick perfumes? Did they know my dirty secret? My palms were sweating and my fingers twitching as I dragged one foot in front of the other to mimic the human walk.

I vividly remember struggling to lift my feet over the curb as I crossed the street. My hand and foot coordination were obsolete by the fifth day of my alcohol bender and I could barely force words out of my thirsty mouth. My body was useless.

An Asian girl walked by, holding her pint-sized yappy dog by the leash, and I asked myself: How does this girl function sober? How can she perform daily tasks without being liquored up? She was annoying; I envied her sobriety. The humdrum of ordinary tedious life drove me senseless. When you're deep in addiction you cannot see others normally. I assumed that everyone had a vice; some were just better at hiding it. I was hiding nothing.

As I turned the corner, I reveled in the beauty of the "Open" liquor store sign. I asked the clerk for a pint of Smirnoff. In broken English, he requested my ID. I shoved my hand in my bag and with erratic, trembling fingers, handed him my ID. He said $7.99 and I gave him a five-dollar bill, then proceeded to count out quarters only to realize I was unable to hold the coins, much less use my brain to count them. My hands were so incredibly weak and feeble that I couldn't bend them. My alcohol withdrawal was in full bloom, like a thorny rose, grisly and dangerous. I piled the coins onto the plastic resin countertop and told the clerk to keep the extra as I darted out of the store, prize in hand.

I shuffled into the first public restroom I could find, in Starbucks. I waited impatiently for two people to use the restroom before I could get my fix. I anxiously stood there observing the "normal" people as they exchanged light banter. These people annoyed me. They were uninteresting and predictable, like prototypes. They had manners, were polite, and were considerate of others. I lacked consideration for even myself.

As I barricaded myself into the unisex bathroom, I didn't even notice the toilet paper that littered the floor, or the drops of urine dried on the toilet seat, as I cracked open the pint of vodka. I put the small red cap on the metal toilet paper holder and swigged the bottle. The poison burned my throat and settled into my stomach like a warm fire. It was soothing. My body was no longer tense, and my limbs slowly came back to life. I needed two more swigs to confidently and successfully screw the red cap back on the bottle. My fingers were no longer trembling and my brain no longer cloudy. Not only was vodka medicine to my aching body, but it was the cure for my indignation with society. Suddenly the world, and the people in it, were my friends. They were no longer ordinary and boring; they were intriguing.

I crumpled up the small brown paper bag, discarding the evidence into the small metal trashcan that was hanging on the wall. I then looked in the tarnished mirror. My eyebrows hadn't been plucked in weeks and my eyeliner haphazardly painted my face. My eyes were glossed over, and my hair was unbrushed, thrown on top of my head to disguise the knots and tangles. I needed that alcohol before I could look in the mirror. What I saw looking back at me was a girl in distress. Her eyes were empty yet filled with the joy of a child on Christmas morning. That little bottle had the magic to transform my mentality. It gave me the confidence to strut out of that small bathroom and endure my day.

The next stop was the bodega next door. As I walked my chipper self into the deli, I politely greeted the regular guys behind the counter. The Smirnoff was hitting my senses and I was becoming increasingly hungry and eager. Food excited me. Food *and* alcohol intoxicated me. The combination was my reason for living. I stood in front of the dessert display and my mind wandered into a trance. The layers of frosting and sugary cakes and colorful sprinkles consumed me. I ended up with a slice of red velvet cake, a vanilla cupcake, a BLT sandwich, and a Vitamin Zero flavored water to wash down the poison.

As I smugly walked back to my apartment, I no longer felt disdain for those ordinary people among me. I felt normal. I could walk over a curb without losing my balance, and most importantly I could carry my bag of food and alcohol without losing grip on my fingers. I felt human again.

One block from my apartment, my oversized Juicy Couture velour track pants ruined my buzz. I tripped on the lengthy bottoms and face-planted into the gritty,

Manhattan sidewalk, littered with cigarette butts and dried gum. My embarrassment was overshadowed by my fierce yearning to get home and drink more. A courteous, attractive young man grabbed my hand and gently helped me off the ground. If I were sober, I would have anticipated a respectful pass from this good-looking young man, who appeared to be in the same age range. He was in my league; we were both easy on the eyes. We would have made a cute couple; the next logical step would have been a number exchange. Unfortunately, I was already in a relationship with alcohol. We were in a long-term relationship, going on five years. But this man never asked for my number, not even my name. He could probably smell the vodka oozing from my pores. I brushed myself off and proceeded home.

The hole in my right pant leg had not phased me. It reminded me of the journey that I had embarked on amidst my full-blown withdrawal. I was a warrior. I felt like Armstrong, like I had triumphantly made it to the moon and back. I was also a hero. My body had been begging for vodka and I complied. I was home, in my dark, cluttered apartment, with my shiny bottle of cheap vodka. I felt accomplished; I felt complete.

I cleared a spot on the floor, pushing clothes and food bags aside. I made a little spot where I would rot for the next seven hours. The small, cleared-away space on the floor was comforting. It was my little nest. I turned on the TV to watch the Food Network and sipped my vodka straight out of a coffee cup that my grandmother had given me that read "Best Granddaughter." The more I sipped, the more that phrase rang true. In my head, I became prettier, smarter, and even funnier. As an alcoholic, I called this phase one, which entails the initial rush. The buzz of the first few drinks was incredible. I began texting my friends and family as normal people did, minus the booze. I became the granddaughter that lived up to my coffee mug. My family back home in Florida had no idea I was on a full-fledged bender. I was in between bartending jobs and was in limbo with life in general.

Phase two involved satisfying my hunger pangs. Alcohol elevated my hunger to a level where food tasted explosive. Drinking also fed the beast, which was my bulimia. Alcohol expanded my stomach capacity and amplified my cravings. Once I started eating, I could not stop. I was powerless.

As I devoured the deli food, I made a conscious effort to intermittently chug my Vitamin Water. This simple action would guarantee an easy purge. Once finished, I migrated to the kitchen, where I devoured the residual junk of last night's takeout. I could not breathe. My stomach was so full that I felt dull pains in my entire midsection. I looked in the mirror and pretended like I was five months pregnant. I rubbed my belly as to mimic my happily pregnant friends that I stalked on Facebook. I got lost in the moment. The fantasy of an entirely different life preoccupied my mind. When I snapped back into reality, I panicked.

I ran to the bathroom before any more food could be digested. I wrapped my arms around the toilet bowl and cathartically purged the two thousand calories that I had consumed minutes earlier. Maybe the red velvet cake wasn't the best idea, but it came up easy and hadn't yet acquired the taste of bile. The red toilet water was traumatizing but not offensive enough to quit. As I stood up, I felt a rush of adrenaline. I no longer felt like a disgusting slob. All evidence of my piggish behavior was flushed down into the endless web of sewer pipes, gone forever. My depravities felt cleansed after a purge. I felt revitalized.

Immediately after eradicating my sins, I grabbed the Smirnoff and gulped straight from the plastic bottle. The burn felt pleasant and invigorating in my empty stomach. I felt a jolt, a joyous kick in the stomach. I could visualize my stomach absorbing the alcohol like a sponge on water. Only the sponge was my stomach, and the water was poison.

Alcohol was my vice and my closest friend. It wreaked havoc on my life yet stabilized my mind. It ignited a fire inside of my soul and simultaneously eased my anxiety. Alcohol was the devil and, when consumed, made me feel like an angel. It gave me wings that allowed me to fly high—high into a delusion that fed my twisted identity. That's what drugs do. They give you wings until you drown, suffocate, or burn.

This is my story that led me to this darkness. As I sat on my floor Indian-style, I asked myself: How did I get here? How did my desire for escaping reality become my reality? It was a simple question that haunted my mere existence.

How did my life as a beautiful girl with a college degree and an effervescent personality become a train wreck?

I became preoccupied with chasing things that I thought would bring me happiness. Behind each controversial decision that my twisted mind made was a craving of some sort. My insatiability in every aspect of my life nearly ruined me. *Enough* is a word that I never used. I was never satisfied.

CHAPTER 2

Cigar Smoke and Mirrors

My earliest memories involve cigar smoke and empty beer cans that clinked as I took out the garbage. My childhood wasn't terrible; it was just chaotic—as most adults would describe their upbringing. I cannot embellish a drawn-out saga that answers the age-old question as to how I became an alcoholic. I wasn't abused or sexually molested and wasn't raised in a one-bedroom apartment with no running water. My childhood wasn't all discouraging, and I certainly cannot link my addictions to a specific event or influential person. I feel like my alcoholism was always in me, dormant and silent. Like an unlit match covered in gasoline. If I played with fire, I went up in flames. The moment I fed the dragon, all hell broke loose.

It probably wasn't the healthiest facet of my childhood to see my father down a twelve-pack of Coors Light every night, but it wasn't the straw that broke the camel's back.

For one thing, my mother did an exceptional job of ensuring that her three children grew up in the most "normal" environment, considering the circumstances of alcohol always being present in the home at all hours of the day. She dedicated almost thirteen years of her life covering up my father's failures, a direct result of his disease. Although an expert at crisis control, it took her until her late forties to realize she could not fix people, particularly people as sick as my father.

My mom was an overweight, blonde firecracker. She was exceptionally skilled at producing small talk with strangers. Her colorful muumuu dresses matched her vibrant personality. She was insecure with her body and utilized food for comfort. My dad provided no comfort or emotional security. He was a man of few emotions. Compassion was not one of those sentiments. His red-tinted skin color matched his anger. Besides the cigar smoke, he always had a distinctive smell to him. It resembled a sweet, fermented, chemical aroma. Anyone who grew up with an alcoholic parent can identify this odor. My dad's odor was complemented by a sizable beer belly. I remember my best friend's mom joking about beer bellies; my dad's belly was not a joke. It was a symptom of his alcoholism.

My dad's involvement in my early life consisted of shouting and reprimanding me when I did something as simple as chewing on my shirt collar, which I did out of nervousness. He would get angry at me for picking up a toy in Walmart or using the wrong word in a sentence. Let's just say, it was extremely easy to annoy and irritate my dad.

As a result, I was constantly second-guessing myself and making sure I was perfect in everything that I executed. I never strived for good; I strived for excellent. There were times when excellent still felt unworthy.

I know my dad loved me unconditionally; he just didn't know how to express himself. His alcoholism had stripped him of any organic emotions. When a normal person feels sad or disappointed, they process and manage those emotions. When an alcoholic feels any ounce of pain, they drink alcohol. This numbs and suppresses the emotional discomfort. The alcohol acts as a Band-Aid. It is a temporary solution to an ongoing problem. The presence of alcohol stunts the healing process and pain is temporarily suppressed. This agony and anger are like a pot of soup. The steam builds up, boils over, and burns. This method always leads to a volcanic explosion. My dad was a volcano that was constantly erupting. My twin sister, my brother, and I were the innocent village people. My mom played the Jolly Green Giant, attempting to smother the hazardous lava with a giant fire extinguisher.

My dad did the best that he could with the cards that he was dealt. My dad spoke little about his childhood, but I could imagine it wasn't idyllic. There were deep cracks in his past and I never expected him to be perfect; I just expected him to do the best that he could. And, that's exactly what he did.

My mom would usually exclude my dad from school functions, vacations, and social gatherings because of his temper. It was like walking on eggshells every time he was in our presence. It was Dad versus Mom and her three children. We weren't a unit; we were hardly a team. When my dad was absent, Mom was outgoing and social. She impressed strangers with her perfectly white smile and charming demeanor. I definitely got my bubbly personality from my mom. She could start a conversation with a wall—that's how eager she was to converse with anybody who would engage.

I blame my mom for the anxiety that I bear whenever I have to make a phone call or get down to the bottom of a situation. She took the reins in every situation and performed those things for me. Even to this day, she talks before I even get a chance to say the first word. She was so accustomed to covering my dad's tracks that she became a "fixer." She fixed everything; she even thought she could fix my dad. Whenever one of her three kids needed something, she was the first person in line. She hired the attorney for my brother's DUI, bailed my sister and me out of jail, and even bailed my dad out of jail when he was pulled over with a beer in his cupholder driving home from an Orlando Magic basketball game. Mom was the classic protector. She was the family's guardian angel. She empowered and enabled.

As a child, I didn't understand alcoholism. I remember my dad getting wasted at my art fair and wondering why he was acting so bizarre. He was literally the only dad holding a Coors Light. All of my friends' parents were drinking iced teas and homemade lemonade. I thought his alcohol consumption was normal. At this art fair, my dad was smoking a cigar and drinking beer, which troubled the lady who was in charge of the crafts booth. This disgruntled, heavyset woman with a raspy voice was in a full-fledged quarrel with my intoxicated father. Then there was my mom, discretely spitting words out of her mouth in an attempt to hush my dad. She forcefully grabbed his arm and started dragging him to the car. Flailing and cursing, he flicked his turd-like cigar butt into the bushes that were decorated with multi-colored Christmas lights and ornaments. The car ride home was pure torture. You could cut the tension with a knife. My parents were taming their frustration with one another and waiting until we got home to rip each other's heads off.

When the forest green Dodge Caravan screeched to a halt in the driveway, we slid open the doors and scurried into the house like scattering deer who'd been spooked. My older brother scampered to his room, which was near the garage, while my sister and I beelined to our rooms toward the back of the house. My mom had this look in her eyes of sheer disappointment. Using only her eyes, she signaled my dad to head straight to their bedroom. He wasn't even allowed to stop at the fridge for a cold one. Once everyone was in their designated rooms, my parents launched their routine bickering.

A normal child would drown out their vexatious voices with loud music or TV. I sat motionless with my ear pressed up against my wood-paneled wall, making out the words they were spitting, gauging the severity of the argument. I listened intently for the "D" word—

When children are byproducts of broken homes, it's rare that they share an equal affinity for both parents. That's just the nature of the beast. Although my dad loved me, I felt like his addiction produced a wedge. I remember being a child and writing letters to my dad begging him to quit smoking. Even before the divorce, I felt the pain of my father's choices. He was there financially while my mom offered a majority of the emotional support.

My mom was a go-getter. As a child I worshipped her. In my eyes, my father was the "bad guy" and my mom played the hero in every plotline of my life. Looking back on this dynamic, it backfired on every level. When my parents divorced when I was thirteen, I developed an anger toward my father that would manifest in various ways throughout my adulthood. Anger was another common theme throughout my life. I'm not sure if it was an inherited trait that I had acquired from my dad or if it was an environmental adaptation directly related to a turbulent childhood. My dad modeled how to treat people and I reproduced his behavior. I didn't know any different. My mom, on the other hand, accepted the emotional abuse. She tolerated the subpar treatment from her spouse. Her insecurities reminded her that she deserved this mediocracy. After all, she was married to this man—till death do us part. Through thick and thin, she weathered the storm.

I remember my mom trying to get my dad to quit drinking. It was a constant battle. Knowing what I know now about the disease of alcoholism, it seemed foolish of her. The battle wasn't between her and my father; it was between her and his alcoholism. Taking the beer out of the equation would've have been fruitless; the drinking was a symptom of my dad's issues, which stemmed from a bumpy childhood. It was solely a coping mechanism. Learning how to process emotions would have been the ideal solution.

School was always my priority. My scholarly achievements distracted me from home life and certainly kept my dad at bay from any disappointment that would lead to frustration. I never wanted to see red in my dad's eyes. I would do anything to avoid poking the bear, especially when the bear was drunk. My dad's irritation was elevated during the day; this was before he had his first beer. He was prickly, cantankerous, and irritable before noon. By nightfall, he was half in the bag. This was a crapshoot. His alcohol-induced bipolarity was a scenario I could never predict. Either way, by the tail end of the night, he was usually arguing with my mom, threatening to leave for the night. Thirty minutes later I could see his aqua blue Kia squeal away into the night as a plume of dust would linger on the dirt road. The house finally seemed so peaceful. The chaos turned into the muffled cries leaking from my parents' bathroom. I knew my mom was sobbing but she did an adequate job at masking her wailing and weeping with soiled tissues held closely to her mouth.

I wanted to be perfect. I wanted to make the best grades, I wanted to be the best softball player, and I wanted to be the best daughter. In my eyes, my dad reinvented a quote: "Perfection, not progress." His persistent criticism made me desperate to avoid even the tiniest of mistakes. This desire for perfection would backfire as I evolved into adulthood. I was in gifted; all through middle school and high school, I felt like I was above the other students who were in honors or regular classes. Although I wasn't the popular cheerleader with countless friends, I was smarter and better than them. At least that is what I told myself to feel better about who I was as a girl. The attention that I received for academics was enough to satisfy my desire for perfection.

My identical twin sister would bear more of the burden of my dad's wrath. She was the introverted sister. She was delicate, perceptive, and relatively more anxious. These qualities became exacerbated after my parents divorced when we were thirteen. It was the summer of 2003 during a trip with our dad. We were visiting his family in Buffalo, New York, when my sister and I made the collective decision to lose our baby fat. My dad consistently made an effort to point out every flaw of ours, he was unsparing. Nothing slid under his radar including our gradual weight gain over the years.

When we initially started losing weight, my sister lost it at a more rapid rate. I lost maybe a couple pounds. By the end of the summer she was down at least twenty. I couldn't understand this discrepancy; we were basically clones of one another. We ate synonymously, we exercised consistently, yet our bodies looked like opposites of each other. We were identical twins; for thirteen years our bodies had been duplicates, indistinguishable. This overturned and agitated me. Throughout our whole existence, we had shared one rare identity. We were a doublet, a team, a force to be reckoned with. Now I felt like she wanted nothing to do with me. She wanted her own identity.

Not long after the Buffalo trip my sister, our best friend Evie, and I traveled to Ohio to visit my grandparents. By this point, my sister was already exhibiting abnormal signs of isolation. Our trio was askew. My sister had retracted and became disengaged with Evie and me. She became preoccupied with food and exercise. She also displayed volatility and agitation, particularly after eating a meal.

There was one night that Evie and I wanted to go to an old-fashioned drive-in movie. We had to convince Erica to come along. She wanted to hang back and exclude herself from our festivities. Why would she choose to stay home with our eighty-year-old grandparents who spent their evening reading the newspaper and watching reruns of old game shows? We bribed her to come along by mentioning that we would make a pit stop at Dairy Queen. Her ears perked up like a dog and she was sold.

At the Queen, she aggressively ordered an extra-large blizzard with Oreos, cheesecake, and cookie dough. I was impressed yet confounded. Perhaps this treat would add a few extra pounds to her astoundingly tiny body. I was ready to force-feed her.

By the time we reached the drive-in movie she had inhaled the entire Blizzard. Her stomach was visibly protruding, and she started complaining of pain and bloating. She became angry, irritable, and prickly. She started squirming in her seat like a child trying to wriggle out of a car seat. She said that she "had to pee" really bad and urgently needed a toilet, but we were at a drive-in movie; there were no restrooms. Sheer panic engrossed her fragile body. We told her to pop a squat in the woods, which was few steps away from our 1995 Ford truck. She scoffed, rolled her eyes, and shot down the idea. She clearly didn't need to go *that* bad.

Looking back on the events of that night, I bet she was looking for a toilet to puke in. Once she realized her lack of opportunity to dispose of the one thousand calories she had eaten, she became angry and hostile. She sat through the entire movie, digesting the food. This was a bulimic's worst nightmare.

I sensed a competitive nature oozing from my sister. We used to be on the same team, and now she wanted to play solo. She made certain her grades were higher, projects were better, and sports were played harder. I knew this wasn't a direct attack on me but a product of her Type A personality. As much as this new mentality distracted me, I didn't respond or react, externally at least. I wanted her to make better grades and run faster in track because I didn't want her to feel defeated. She was the sensitive twin and I couldn't bear to witness her distraught. My role in the duo was the social one, while she was the perfectionist with the perfect grades. I recognized and accepted my place and I stayed in my lane.

I remember it was sophomore year when my sister and I were enrolled in AP (advanced placement) world history. The class proved incredibly challenging; even the top students struggled to pull a B+, including my sister. It was the final test to determine how many college credits we would receive based on a score from one to five. For three weeks we frantically checked the mailbox for the large white envelopes from the College Board that housed the prized results. When the envelopes finally arrived at our residence, we frantically ripped them open like they were birthday cards with wads of cash. I noticed my sister shriek in terror as she read the giant number 3 smack dab in the center of the page. She was devastated. Based on her reaction, I thought she'd scored a 0.

When I directed my eyeballs downward toward my own results, I noticed a giant 4 staring back at me. I swiftly crumpled up the coveted piece of flimsy paper and tossed it directly into the trash. For a split-second, Erica forgot about her ordeal and asked me the dreaded question, "What did you get?" In a shaky, cracked voice I said, "I got a 3 also." She took a deep sigh of relief, then continued to sob. I couldn't do it. I couldn't divulge the shocking revelation. I couldn't do that to my sister. I couldn't break the potentially devastating news to my broken and delicate twin. She was not in the right frame of mind to comprehend such outrageous intel. She was too sensitive to handle the possibility that I could be potentially smarter than her. It was not possible.

That same year, my mom tapped me on the shoulder with this look of transparent dysphoria and panic. My mom was always translucent. She wore her emotions on her sleeve. This provoked me for many years, but as an adult I have learned to appreciate and respect the quality of transparency. She was powerless in her ability to uphold a poker face. She was enthusiastic, devout, and, most importantly, loving. Her transparency was a product of her passion.

On this morning, my mom wore a look on her face that was foreign to me. She handed me a journal that she had discovered while cleaning my sister's room. Why she was cleaning my sister's already immaculate and tidy room remains a mystery to this day. She flipped the pages with her frantic hand to a page that read something like this: "Everyone has a vice. Everyone has an addiction. You're not alone. Addictions come and go. They fade out and they disappear. You need this addiction now. It's a time in your life that you need this to get through things. Throwing up is not that bad."

The rest of the journal pages consisted of daily summations of caloric intake, broken down to each morsel of food. It looked something like this:

Monday
Apple: 50 calories
2 crackers: 35 calories
2 sips of nonfat milk: 25 calories
3 stalks of celery: 20 calories
TOTAL: 130 calories

This devastated and broke my mom. This was the first indication of addiction passed down to her offspring. We come from a legacy of alcoholics and essentially a lineage of mental health obstacles that include food addiction, anxiety, agoraphobia, alcoholism, and depression. No parent envisions that their child will become an addict. Even if it's hereditarily passed down from one generation to another, it's one of those scenarios where we assume that the legacy will break in relation to our own children. It is legitimately a form of torture to witness your children suffer with self-destructive thoughts and compulsive behaviors.

I, on the other hand, felt relieved. All my questions had been answered in an uncomplicated and stupid journal. The unambiguous interpretation for her dramatic weight loss was a diabolical one. She was restricting her caloric intake while concurrently purging the regular, calorific food that she did consume. How does a parent process this intel? How does a child adopt such self-destructive behaviors at such a delicate age? My heart was broken. Our relationship would never be the same.

My sister's eating disorder would follow her through every nook and cranny of her life, and eventually mine. The disease would rear its ugly head, inadvertently and recurrently. There were moments in life where it was dormant; she was asymptomatic. Then there were the hospitalizations, the heart palpitations, the hidden bags of vomit underneath the bed, all succeeded by a thirty- to ninety-day stint in an eating disorder treatment facility.

The comments that were unintentionally generated from my father throughout our formative years proved destructive. Parents don't understand that even seemingly trivial criticisms are detrimental to a child's self-worth. I remember feeling constant guilt and dissatisfaction through those years. I was the perfect child, yet I was being critiqued for the way that I washed the dog or the way that I cooked a potato. I was walking on eggshells twenty-four hours a day, seven days a week. These feelings of inadequacy perpetuated into every aspect of my life. I outperformed and overkilled every undertaking. This ensured me that I wouldn't feel guilty for not giving it my all. I know my sister felt the same way.

Dieting was an avenue that she took to control her environment. It was the one aspect of her life that she could regulate. It gave her a sense of power in a household dominated by an alcoholic patriarch. Her eating disorder was her pride and joy. She felt accomplished. She had not an ounce of fat on her tiny five-foot-two frame. For every pound of fat that was shed was a flaw that was removed. She felt accomplished and perfect.

The weight on her body represented baggage. It symbolized every undesirable remark from my father and every invasive thought from her own mind. When this physical weight was purged, she felt mentally enlightened. The weight of any insecurities was lifted off her shoulders. Ironically, the disease of her eating disorder conceived even more angst within her restless mind. Even though she had a flawless body with zero fat, she embodied zero confidence.

My teen years were astonishingly substantial and steady. Unlike my sister, I loved my body. I cultivated and protected my youth and my overall health. I formed sound decisions and evaded potentially precarious situations; i.e., sex, alcohol, and drugs. My confidence was unwavering, and my morals were unshakable. When I looked in the mirror, I saw a beautiful, intelligent, playful, and tenacious girl looking back at me. As a human, these are the organic qualities I exhibited while sober and temperate. The instantaneous moment that alcohol kissed my lips, all those alluring qualities were expelled.

Alcohol dimmed the fire in my soul. It broke me. It paralyzed my passion and suffocated my spirit. It modified the person that I strived to be in this world. Alcohol and drugs are truly outlaws to society. They obstruct human originality, anatomically and intellectually. When you look in the mirror, under the influence of drugs or alcohol, the reflection that stares back at you is merely a shell of your organic self.

Was that journal entry that my sister created nearly twenty years ago an age-old sentiment? Does every human suffer from some degree of addiction at one point or another? Does this philosophy excuse certain behaviors, or is it simply a hypothesis designed to make us feel better about our vices?

CHAPTER 3

Shrek Is Not for Kids

College changed everything. I got accepted into the University of Florida, which was a high-achieving institution. This meant that every student was gifted. For once, I felt like an average and mediocre student. It wasn't easy to stand out in this school. I simply wasn't smart enough. My desire for differentiation propelled me toward attention-seeking behavior. I became open-minded and began experimenting with boys and drinking, all while achieving less than average grades.

Before college, I had despised alcohol. I associated my father and his erratic behavior with the penalties of drinking. My father was like a bad advertisement for alcohol. I assumed that if I drank any alcohol at all, that I would transform into my critical father. The decision to pick up my first drink during my freshman year was a metamorphic one.

This transformational experience brought me out of my shell. I had been very guarded, rigid, and straight-laced before I met alcohol. Alcohol empowered me. It invented me. I loved the girl that emerged after a couple drinks. My introversion became extroversion. My social constraints became unconstrained, and my silence became laughter. My newfound self was emerging, and I foresaw no impediments. I was a social butterfly. I spread my wings and, eventually, my legs. I became a girl that I wasn't proud of.

My proliferating social circle included the types of boys that I was not accustomed to. I had never really coexisted with males who were sexually motivated. This was new to me; this was uncharted territory. *My body* was uncharted territory. That is, of course, until I became acquainted with alcohol. Alcohol took my virginity. It stole my spirit and my originality. It not only broke my true self, it annihilated it. My mindful, conscientious character transformed into a person I didn't even recognize; yet I yearned to permanently become *that* girl.

That girl that I became was addicted to attention. I craved attention regardless of the toll. I deliberately befriended the fraternities that were less-fortunate looking. I wanted to be the girl who every guy wanted. I wanted to be that femme fatal. In hindsight, I became the *easy* girl who every guy wanted to sleep with but no one wanted to date. I was repulsive.

The fraternity that I preyed on was AEPi. They were the Jewish fraternity at the University of Florida and primarily consisted of nerdy, conservative guys who hardly stood above five feet, five inches tall. They were immature, inexperienced, and relatively new to the party scene. We had *that* in common. They were recently released into the wild after being held in captivity by their demanding, successful parents who were all lawyers and doctors. Their newfound sense of freedom was evident on their wide-eyed faces as they drooled over mediocre girls.

I chased and sought out guys whom I knew wouldn't reject me. I was insecure and self-doubting, yet confident in my ability to attract the attention of this fraternity. This fraternity did me dirty on a night that would disgust even the most seasoned whores.

It was the summer of 2009. I was getting ready to drag my roommate to a party at the AEPi fraternity house. I remember trying on different black dresses. I chose a knit, stretchy dress that barely covered my butt cheeks. I always chose the most provocative outfit in my closet. That was my mode of operation. "Go slutty or go home" was my motto. I was about fifteen pounds overweight but still looked more appealing than the other sorority girls that frequented that frat house on weekends. They were the AEPhi girls who were their equivalents. They were equally "hard on the eyes."

My roommate and I downed three shots each of cotton candy-flavored Pinnacle vodka and then trekked six blocks over to the hideous, unkempt, and outdated house where the infamous party would take place. As I walked in the front door, the smell of fermented beer, moldy wallpaper, and freshly sprayed Axe Spray consumed my senses. I felt a rush of anticipation. I was ready for alcohol to morph me into my alter ego. I was thirsty. This metamorphosis was foreseeable to every eager, unhygienic frat boy in that colossal, malodorous mansion. Everyone knew that after seven shots of crummy vodka and several cups of flat beer, I would become Lady Godiva. By the third game of beer pong, I was flirting with everything that had two eyes and a mouth.

My favorite frat boy was named Dean. I would occasionally get drunk enough to sleep with him but avoided that catastrophe while sober. I had to be blackout drunk to hook up with this guy, and fortunately for him I was always blackout drunk. I was unequivocally not attracted to him. He reminded me of Shrek by the shape of his head and the way he slouched his shoulders. He had a giant mole right above his lip that was quite distracting because of the hairs that protruded from it. That was the only facial hair he could grow, those three tiny black hairs. I felt sorry for Shrek. Aside from being less than fortunate looking, he had a hearing aid. He could barely hear me shrieking across the AEPi house as I got drunker and drunker. I liked hanging out with him because he always provided me with a dorm-sized refrigerator full of Jack Daniel's. His accommodations were top-notch considering that the rest of his buddies were drinking stale beer. Shrek loved drinking with me. He used me and I used him; it was mutual.

On this night, Shrek swooped in prematurely. He accurately gauged my level of intoxication and took it upon himself to steal me away from the party. I remember walking down the hallway to his room as I began unbuckling my bra strap. I wanted to get this escapade over with so that I could return to the party and continue my attention-seeking behavior. After a fuzzy rendezvous and a couple shots of Jack Daniel's, I returned to the party.

Shortly after, Shrek called it a night, but I was far from throwing in the towel. I was elated that he had made the decision to remain upstairs because, quite frankly, I couldn't stand him. He was creepy and would stare at me with his half-open eyes as I would aggressively flirt with his frat brothers. I was always paranoid that Shrek, hearing aid intact, could eavesdrop on all my raunchy conversations with his friends. His bionic ears freaked me out. What was this cartoon character capable of? I've watched way too many episodes of *Dateline* and *Forensic Files*, and quite frankly, this kid resembled the creep next door who stole your panties straight out of the bottom drawer.

As the night progressed, my memory became loose and eventually nonexistent. The last thing I vividly remember is walking in on one of the frat boys taking a dump in one of bathroom stalls on the second floor. I quickly slammed the door shut as I squealed in a high-pitched voice, "Ooops, sorry!" The smell crawling out of that stall was unforgettable, unlike the night that was about to unfold. Even though I couldn't remember a thing, this night was memorable to every fraternity on campus and would inevitably devastate my already smeared and shaky reputation.

I returned to a group of boys playing cards downstairs where I eagerly rehearsed the humorous event that had happened minutes earlier. The last and final memory I had is taking a double shot of bourbon. This shot charred my raw, cracked throat; that was the drink that would take me over the edge. I went from being a functioning human to a rag doll that could barely hold myself up. My limbs became powerless and inert while my head bobbed from side to side like a bobblehead. I was just as pathetic as a cheap plastic toy. My brain function went from seven to zero in less than ten seconds. I could no longer pronounce words, much less make out a full sentence. I tried to focus my eyes on the guys who were standing around me, but my eyes kept rolling back into my head. I wanted to stay present, alert, and alive but the alcohol had different plans for me. I was fading and there was nothing I could do about it. The party was thinning out, and the mood turned thick. I was gone.

I woke up the next morning and my head was spinning. I was disappointed that I was in Shrek's undesirable bed. I was laying on top of his off-white colored comforter, wearing nothing but an oversized t-shirt. I loathed the feeling of not wearing panties in bed. I felt clammy and could feel my thighs kissing. I was somewhat alleviated when I realized I had slept on top of the covers. I immediately visualized what lived and laid dormant inside of Shrek's unwashed sheets. Dirt, grime, and venereal diseases were among them. I felt dirty, but not from the sheets. Realistically, I was among the dirt in those sheets; I was a piece of dirt. I felt like scum. I felt repulsive. I knew that if I took a shot of alcohol, I would feel worthy again.

Those sheets were no better than me. They wore the wear-and-tear of many scandalous and distasteful nights. They were grody and overworked. They needed a hefty, thorough wash, just as I needed a comprehensive cleanse. I felt sorry for Shrek's sheets and the horrifying things they had to witness. They were used and recycled, just like I was the night before.

I could feel Shrek breathing on me. I felt every inhale and exhale. It angered me. Just as I was planning my escape maneuver, Shrek rolled over like an Italian sausage on a sizzling hot pan. His attempt at a morning acknowledgment consisted of a moist, slobbery kiss on the cheek. His breath smelled like mothballs, which made me want to hurl. In fact, I did hurl. I ran to the stalls across the hall and projectile vomited cheap vodka and sour beer. I felt more disgusting than hundred-year-old sheets that have never been washed.

When I returned to Shrek's den, he proceeded to stick his hand where it didn't belong. I was sick with a head-thumping, room-turning kind of hungover. I wanted to die. I wanted to take Shrek's hand and break it. I wanted all of his bones to shatter. I was angry.

I was also in a complete daze. I was not myself. I felt vodka oozing from my pores. I was completely out of reality and still half drunk. I felt like I was in purgatory. I was halfway between feeling drunk and feeling sober. I did not want to feel sober because that would make me feel even more disgusted with myself. If I were to have an "out of body" experience, I would be looking down in repugnance. I would notice details that I couldn't recognize if I weren't half in the bag. I would see the tiny ants that collected near the crumbs on Shrek's desk. I would notice the stains on Shrek's sheets that resembled dry yogurt. I would notice the undisturbed dust that was two inches thick on Shrek's nightstand. I would notice the smell of a sweaty jockstrap. I would even notice the tiny mold that dotted the cheese that I was munching on the night before.

Fortunately, I was not in my right mind. My Type A, perfectionist self was altered. My body and my mind needed an exorcism. I was dominated by this evil spirit. This literal "spirit" was named vodka. I needed Jesus. I needed someone to purge this evil that was overcoming my poor, incapacitated body.

What was I hiding from? Why did I find it necessary to become this altered self? Why was this disgusting predicament okay with me? Why would I rather wake up in Shrek's bed than wake up in my own, feeling sober and normal? Why was I not okay feeling normal? These questions were never rendered during this period of time in my life. I never asked myself why. I thought that these were the customary college catastrophes. These mornings occurred long before the term "alcoholic" even grazed my tongue. This was just college; that's what everybody did. Sadly, the events that were about to unfold were far from college shenanigans.

By the time I got home from Shrek's lair, I was exhausted. I laid in my bed and allowed my head to spin off into la-la land. My dreams were warped and twisted, just like my mind. I woke up nineteen hours later and it was Monday, the most cringeworthy day of the week. It was the day that partying and drinking were not acceptable. It was the day that the rest of world would resume their working existence. Lawyers buttoned up their suits and jumped in their Audis. Nurses put on their scrubs and fueled up with a bowl of oatmeal. The graveyard shifters were just arriving home and unwinding on the couch. I put on my spandex and baggy t-shirt and dragged myself out of my house. I was agitated, distraught, and angry that the weekend had come to an end.

I did not want to be normal. I was never able to accept the reality that I had lived a productive life during the week. I wanted my life to be a never-ending party. I wondered how people woke up so early for work almost every day. I did not understand their dedication and habitual natures. My only habit-forming behaviors were negative in nature. I was diseased.

I raced out the door to meet my friend Jessie at the Reitz Center Food Court. Saturday night's episode vaguely replayed in my head. I was wondering why Jessie was so adamant in meeting with me on this uninteresting, stale afternoon. The thought that I had done something incredibly stupid on Saturday night crossed my mind, as it always had. I had no inkling that I was about to hear a story that would be unsuitable for the faint of heart. The story that

Jessie would tell would be scandalous, unconvincing, and downright nauseating. It was the scene of a sleazy, low-budget independent film. It was truly unbelievable, even to me, the protagonist of the scene.

Jessie, who was hooking up with the house manager of the AEPi fraternity house, extended details of the events that had taken place on Saturday night. "Events that took place" is a euphemism for "Alcohol-induced disgusting behavior." I was just about to bite into my Subway sub when she explained that I had participated in physical engagements with multiple guys two nights prior. Although a first, that info was not overly heinous or shocking. I was surprisingly okay and composed as I took my second bite from my six-inch turkey sub. Then, Jessie gave me the distasteful details about each encounter and the crisis that transpired. It shook me to the core. The two bites I had taken from my sub were about to be regurgitated. All the blood rushed out of my head. My face turned white and my heart stopped beating for three seconds. I was speechless, sober, and shocked.

When my heart started beating again, it didn't just beat, it raced. I could feel it pumping. It was working overtime to supply blood to my body that was in shock. I couldn't speak, I couldn't think, I couldn't even digest the half-eaten sub that I had consumed minutes earlier.

Jessie's boy-toy had intel that he voluntarily shared with her. He had witnessed the entire sequence of events from Saturday night. He then wrote a blog about every explicit detail that manifested from my drunken escapade.

He then sent the blog via mass email to every single fraternity on the List Serv. Therefore, every guy who was in a fraternity at the University of Florida was now informed that a blonde girl, named Brittany, was a complete whore. I was not the only star of the show. Apparently, another wasted girl and a bottle of Patron had made an appearance. The blog also incorporated details such as the color of my underwear and the scope of my landing strip. I was petrified.

Petrified was an understatement. How could I survive this type of indecent exposure? My mind started racing while Jessie kept reassuring me that "everything is going to be okay." I could see it in her eyes that she was blatantly lying. It was the equivalent of telling someone who just had their sex tape leaked that "it wasn't that big of a deal." The only thing missing from this whole story is a video. Fortunately, a video never surfaced.

As I sat at that small table in front of the Subway sign, I began to feel my heart beating, my blood boiling, and my overall adrenaline shoot through the roof. I felt tears running down my face and the pressure building up from the anger that I was experiencing. There was, of course, anger for the perverts who took advantage of my lifeless, incoherent body, but there was also a special kind of anger for myself and my own behavior. How did this happen? I used to be the girl who wouldn't even go near alcohol. I was the girl proud of my virginity and would certainly never waste a second on a dud. These boys were all duds.

That's the incredible thing about alcohol. It changes who you are as a human being. It completely hijacks your morals and your identity. It drowns the voices in your head that remind you that something is a bad idea. It hushes your conscience and feeds your rebellion. It releases the dragon inside your soul. My quiet, rigid, boring persona transformed into a spunky, gregarious, and provocative entity. For the first time in my life, I craved all eyes on me. I was hungry for attention, and alcohol was the antidote.

This scandalous blog was pivotal in my alcoholic history. It was my defining moment. It solidified my lust for any form of attention. As disgusting as I was with myself, I relished in the fact that everyone was talking about me. I felt famous. I felt important.

Why did I crave this feeling of importance at any cost? Was it some inadequacy from childhood that lingered into my adulthood? That constant need and desire to gratify and fulfill your parents' expectations is powerful. We underestimate the torture children endure by feeling like they're not good enough. This inability to meet expectations as children manifests into maladaptive behaviors as adults.

Fear was the driving force that propelled me through success as a child. I never wanted to disappoint my dad and I continued to work hard to make my mom proud. The second I stepped foot onto the University of Florida campus I felt the weight of all expectations tumble off my shoulders. My dad was essentially out of the picture at this point. He was deep into his alcohol addiction with his new wife. Meanwhile, my alcoholic career was in its infancy stage. Alcoholic inception was being rooted. These roots would grow deep and thick. They would become thirsty, mangled, and twisted. These were the roots of a prickly cactus. This cactus would endure many years of torture from the hot sun. It would scare off any beacon of success and health. Its capacity to survive in such callous conditions was remarkable. The hot sun delineates the beatings my body suffered from gallons and gallons of alcohol.

Alcohol is perceived as poison to the human body and the brain. The liver processes the poison in an incredible attempt to rid and cleanse the body. The liver works in overdrive and regenerates to compensate for the compromised state that alcohol induces. The body is meant to be a well-oiled machine. If alcohol is consistently tainting the machinery, those parts become rusty. Once this degeneration begins, there's no turning back. You can't "undo" all those years of alcohol poisoning. The only way to combat this erosion is to quit drinking before your body fails. All for what? A decade of partying and numbing out?

The pain of addiction spans far beyond the struggle to gain sobriety. The body inevitably carries the weight of all those years of abuse. Of course, the body bounces back, but only to a certain degree. At the ripe age of twenty-eight, I would make a vow to take care of my body, my mind, and my organs so that they could withstand and endure one hundred-plus years of life on this earth. If we ignore the damage we do *today*, then *tomorrow* is going to be a scary fucking day.

CHAPTER 4

A Drunken Situation

Attention-seeking behavior was my trademark and my mode of operation throughout college. I had developed an appetite for chaos and an insatiable lust for fame. I cultivated an itch for negative attention; it was better than no attention at all. This story begins in the summer between junior and senior year of college, approximately one year after the fraternity scandal. This was a hall of fame moment. The second most defining moment of my drinking career.

My twin sister was fresh out of rehab. This would be her third stint in treatment for her debilitating eating disorder. We had exhilarating adventures planned for the summer. We were set to study abroad with UF's College of Journalism and Communications in Florence, Italy. I literally scooped my twin sister up from the rehab doorsteps and together we hopped on a flight to Rome.

My sister was fragile and delicate. She had recently restored most of her weight back from an eating disorder that had nearly killed her. Despite this fragility and vulnerability, I stuffed my hesitations deep inside my rapidly flowing mind. All skepticism and angst were left behind in the United States. We were reunited and it felt glorious. We were a duo; we were unstoppable and rebellious. We refused to listen to anyone, not even each other. Our ebullient personalities were a force to be reckoned with. We complemented each other. I was unrestrained and fearless. My sister was cautious and intelligent. Together, we lit up a room.

The second we arrived in Florence, we wasted no time exploring the city and the cocktails. We pretended to be normal college kids. We had convinced ourselves that we drank in decent moderation alongside our classmates. Nothing seemed completely out of the ordinary at this juncture of my alcoholic career. I exhibited signs of alcoholism, but nothing I couldn't chalk up to stereotypical college shenanigans.

The first night abroad was a tragic one. It was an alcoholic blunder that I had made many times before. My sister and I went over to our classmate's apartment for a little party on the opposite side of Florence. At around 9 p.m. we arrived at the apartment, where people were playing flip cup, beer pong, and other quintessential college drinking games. We brought the party to Florence. This was the first time my sister and I had partied together in over three months. We were twinning. We were throwing back cheap wine and mocking our classmates who were in bed by 8 p.m. We had the entire apartment roaring with laughter.

We carried the party into the wee hours of the night. The last memory I retained was drinking a tall boy followed by a shot of gin. I hated gin. My sister had weaseled her way into someone's bedroom and was snugly sleeping off the booze. I had managed to pass out on this maroon-colored, Italian upholstered bench chair that was peculiarly positioned in the kitchen.

When I woke up, my yellow and gray striped dress was bunched up near my waist. My hair was enmeshed in my beaded necklace, and my head was pounding faster than a runner on pavement. I scanned the vacant room and released a deep sigh. I readjusted my legs and noticed that the bottom of my dress was damp. I released another deeper sigh. I instantaneously threw myself off the bench to properly identify the unsightly wet spot that graced the center of this ambiguous piece of furniture. My heart started pounding faster than my spinning head. I had to make moves before my classmates emerged. The stain was unmistakable and unambiguous. I tiptoed out of the squeaking apartment, leaving my sister in the dust.

Two weeks into our studies, the cast of the MTV reality show *Jersey Shore* began filming season four. The cast, the crew, and the paparazzi completely uprooted the low-key and charming city. Florence became mayhem. *Jersey Shore* was flowing out of everyone's mouth. The show, and its boisterous cast members, was the talk of the town. People were captivated by the quarrelsome and unruly bunch.

They lacked class, humility, and respect. Regardless, I wanted to meet them.

It was a Sunday night and we were finishing up gnocchi, margarita pizza, and a bottle of Chianti. The half bottle of wine that I drank wasn't enough. I was still thirsty. I pined for intoxication. One drink was never enough. The moment that I tasted alcohol on my tongue, I longed for more. I loathed the feeling of tipsy. In my mind, it was a half-assed attempt at getting drunk. It was a failure. I would rather be sober than tipsy at all.

Since no one wanted to go out with me on that fateful Sunday night, I flew solo. I walked into the first bar that I saw. I waited at the bar for an Italian native to buy me a drink. Then, I migrated to a table by myself. Literally, five minutes later, I saw three enormous cameras, followed by three bright lights, followed by the entire cast of the reality show *Jersey Shore*. I nervously shifted my body position to mimic an air of confidence. I hastily combed my fingers through my hair and readjusted my bra to accentuate my cleavage.

I made direct eye contact with Mike "The Situation" Sorrentino, one of the stars of the show. He did a modest double-take and proceeded to sit directly next to me. His eyes kept deviating from left to right as if he were admiring all the onlookers. I initiated small talk and instantly realized that this guy was not normal. He could barely cultivate a two-minute conversation without inadvertently complimenting himself. You could tell that he revered himself. He loved his glued-back hair, his beefy muscles, and, of course, his overly bronzed four-pack. He was quite the package. At least he thought so. His eyes bore a blank stare that matched his flaky attitude. His demeanor and his detachment implied that he was in space. He was not on this planet and neither was I.

The Situation was a new and improved version of Shrek. Apparently, I was attracted to these characters. The Situation was the same height as Shrek. The only stark difference between the two was that Shrek was green and The Situation was orange.

The lights, the cameras, and the crowds of people were intoxicating. In that moment, I lost sight of any worries that plagued me. I also lost partial consciousness. I would have to wait three agonizing months until the show aired to witness the details of that first night with The Situation. All I could recall was signing a million pages of consents before I could enter the cast's posh apartment. By the time I finished signing contracts with producers, I was virtually sober.

When I climbed up the wide staircase, a sense of panic overwhelmed me. I was only half drunk and progressively becoming more cognizant of the situation that I was confronting, pun intended. I whispered to myself, "What am I doing?" and "Am I making a mistake?" I knew the answer, but the alcohol reassured me. Alcohol's persuasion was credible and convincing. It had an extraordinary power over my mind when it came to decision-making. In that moment, it pushed me right through those doors into an environment not suitable for a broken girl like me.

On that same night, I felt degraded. I remember laying in Mike's bed for hours waiting for him to return from an argument he was having with Snooki. He was cooking chicken cutlets, smoking cigarettes, and conversing with everyone in the house, while I was sitting in a room with no phone, no TV, and no windows. If this was "real life" I would have stormed my happy ass out of that door with steam coming out of my ears. Instead, I lay there in docility, like a dog. I was obedient and inferior, merely because of his fame.

The Situation gave me explicit instructions to stay in the bed. He made demands, and I followed them. This lack of respect was disgusting. I waited for over an hour. I was a puppet with no self-worth or voice to speak up for myself. He barked at me like a chauvinist. I don't know if it was because I was a female or because I was a regular person, but I feel like that wasn't an uncommon occurrence. I wasn't a celebrity and he knew I was a pushover.

Society perceives famous people as having net worth and value. Therefore, we somewhat worship celebrities. This idolization gives certain famous people an arrogance and an untouchability. Consequently, they feel as if they can behave any way they desire toward others. They are conditioned to feel important. Importance breeds assurance for most celebrities and pretension and vanity for others, particularly reality TV stars.

As an ordinary person, you cannot prepare yourself. I was stuck in a house with a group of celebrities who made me feel like I was the most worthless piece of shit. Snooki proved to be the least reserved. She blatantly called me "ugly," "slut," and "whore." Of course, I chuckled and brushed the harsh words off. What else was there to do? I felt subordinate and powerless. Snooki only confirmed my preconceived notions.

The rest of the cast were demeaning and provoking. They ignored my presence; I got the impression that I was not worth talking to. I was not on their celebrity level. I was not a real person. When I think about those evoked emotions to this day, I get choked up. How can people treat others in such a despicable way? I understand that I put myself in that position, but what I don't understand is the brazen lack of respect for another human being. They were riding high on their horses. I felt uncomfortable, inferior, and worthless. My deepest regret was returning to their house after that first night. If I were sober, I would have cut off all contact and protected myself. If I were sober, I wouldn't have conversed with The Situation and I certainly wouldn't have returned home with him.

Since my appearance on the show, there was one question that I got asked the most: "Was the cast nice to you?" I always answered that question with a lie. "Of course." I was too mortified and confounded to accept the reality that I was not worth a celebrity's time. I was a waste. I was garbage.

The next thing I remember is waking up in the Smoosh Room with Mike tapping me on the shoulder, broadcasting in a cracked voice, "Your cab's downstairs." My head was spinning, and I kept trying to wake up from this tragic yet all-too-realistic nightmare. There were no windows, just cameras that saturated every angle of the room. I unenthusiastically spent the next ten minutes scouring the tiny room for my black and white striped tank top. Mike seemed allayed and slightly less irritated when I found the shirt that he had worked so hard to remove hours earlier. I threw my panties into the pocket of my black, denim shorts and scurried out of the room with my tail in between my legs.

When I got back to our apartment, I plugged my phone in to charge it. When life was restored, I noticed that I had about twenty missed calls from the States. I was worried. Did a family member pass away? Did my cat die? Did I win a seven-day cruise to the Eastern Caribbean? I was exploding with curiosity so I called my friend who was back in Gainesville. The phone rang three times before she picked up. Before she could say anything, I asked her if everything was okay. She responded, "Yes, of course." She asked me if I had seen the news. Obviously, I hadn't seen any news because I was 4,238 miles away from the United States. So, I told her to spill the dirt. And that's exactly what she proceeded to do.

She said she had seen me on TMZ smooching Mike the Situation in front of Florence's most iconic landmark. I couldn't deny it; the proof was in the pictures. I honestly didn't remember kissing him on the streets of Florence probably because I didn't remember walking home. I didn't even remember leaving the club and I certainly didn't remember paparazzi taking photos. I was blacked out. I was paralyzed with fear and anticipation. I felt famous. I was embarrassed and excited at the same time. I was dealing with conflicting emotions.

The next few nights would play out interchangeably. Mike would disclose where to go, and my sister and I would meet him at the club. We didn't realize that when the show aired, they were going to label us as stalkers. The Situation explicitly exposed his location every single night. It's not like we had a GPS strapped to his shoe that allowed us to stalk his movements. This label devastated us.

We partied with the cast for a total of four nights. My sister, who was a virgin at the time, made multiple ill-advised decisions that would shake her integrity for years to come. Alcohol affected her similarly; she went from being this sober and soft-spoken girl to the life of the party. Alcohol rocked her persona and modified her core values.

It was the first time my sister would meet the crew. I got dolled up and threw on one of the three dresses that I had packed for the trip. I kept recycling outfits that, unbeknownst to me, would appear on TV. I was wearing a red and white striped dress that barely covered my butt cheeks, and Erica was sporting a navy-blue dress that was see-through, if you squinted hard enough. We left our apartment and obviously hit up the liquor store, per usual. The clubs that we frequented banned outside liquor, and the drinks inside the club were too expensive for a couple of unemployed college girls.

When you're poor, you become craftier. You manipulate situations in order to save a buck. On this night in question, we hid four airplane bottles of vodka into a compact, feminine pad box. We shoved a pad over the bottles to disguise the precious alcohol. We approached the line and were able to bypass many of our male counterparts. We felt like we were in the United States. We shuffled right through security; they made a modest attempt to scrutinize our belongings. I felt a rush of adrenaline as we both looked at each other with a devious smirk. We were partners in crime. We were thick as thieves. We were two sisters and two alcoholics who were thirsty for a concrete thrill.

When the cast made their appearance, the integral vibe of the club shifted. Strangers were throwing themselves in front of the camera and flocking around the celebrities, who were dressed in tacky and hideous neon colors. I introduced Mike to my sister and the rest was history. He became a wide-eyed kid on Christmas morning. To this day, I'm not sure if it was for the cameras or if he really thought my sister and I would have a threesome with him. Regardless, we made the fool believe that he had a chance with the two of us. There was something magical about being in front of the camera. It was an instantaneous high. The bright lights and the masses of people were intoxicating. These ingredients were a recipe for disaster, especially for an alcoholic.

Alcohol eradicates your inhibitions. It holds your rationality hostage and steals your sanity. Your core, along with your values, becomes nonexistent. Normal people would avoid the tragedy of *Jersey Shore*; the mere thought of being caught dead with these clowns would send the average, rational person running for the hills. When you're an addict, you experience these insatiable cravings; you want more of whatever gives you pleasure. Being in front of the camera was absolutely exhilarating. One appearance wasn't enough. I was thirsty for more. I had never in my life experienced a high like this. It was pure adrenaline. It was *almost* better than alcohol.

On that night, my sister was so wasted that she made out with both Deena and Vinny. I painstakingly witnessed my sister make one of the most scandalous and shocking blunders of her life. I fathomed she was in a blackout. I was right.

Keep in mind, my sister was a perfectionist. She was introverted, soft-spoken, and unassured. She would never in a million years inject herself into such a slippery predicament. She was totally out of her element, and alcohol was the culprit. Alcohol was a deviant. It slithered into our minds and manipulated our levelheaded preset. I knew in my heart that my sister would wholeheartedly regret every aspect of that night. At the same time, I couldn't stop her. Alcohol had already saturated her intelligent brain. For the rest of the night, I lost my sister. She lost herself along with her impeccable reputation.

I could already predict holding my sister's hand as this humiliating episode aired. I pictured her sobbing uncontrollably. She had worked hard to foster her integrity as a woman for twenty-two prolonged years. And, in the blink of an eye, everything shattered.

The reality is, college students party and inevitably make regretful decisions all the time. They wake up the next morning and carry on with their lives. Their drunken mistakes are forever forgotten, buried deep inside the brain.

In *our* unique situation, pun intended, our mistakes were aired for the entire world to see. In a stranger's mind, those few episodes characterized who we were as humans. We were two desperate, drunk girls who were deficient in morality and class. We were trash, just like the clowns who starred on the show. The only difference between us and them: we had collectively $50 to our names, and they had millions. We were suckers; we felt used. This erroneous portrayal would eventually define who I was for the subsequent four years.

Blacking out on national television was scarier than waking up in a stranger's bed the next morning. It is actually ten times worse. You have to sit and stare at a TV watching a drunk person that you don't even recognize. You want to jump through the screen and shake yourself. You want to reverse the alcohol. You beg to go back in time and sip one less vodka and Diet Coke and take six fewer shots of chilled Patron. You yearn for the world to see your true colors shine, in the words of Cyndi Lauper. Except, we weren't shining like a rainbow; we were dark clouds looming over the city of Florence.

The Situation called me at 5 p.m. on a weekday and left me a message reiterating the projected plan for the night. They were either going to Space, which was a disco club in the heart of Firenze, or heading to a quaint bar on the outskirts of the city for a low-key kind of night. He never clarified where to meet him so I took it upon myself to show up at their apartment, something I would never have done if I were sober.

That evening, my sister and I decided to experiment with Absinthe, the botanical liquor that supposedly makes you hallucinate. We went shot for shot with each other. The green color was grossly exhilarating. It was like drinking Beetle Juice. Right before taking my third shot, I imagined myself floating around the city feeling as light as a feather. I hallucinated a tiff with Snooki and even a rendezvous with the Situation. After sobering up, I realized that these were not hallucinations; these were events that actually took place. This was my reality.

I blacked out after a few shots of the absinthe. The last thing I remembered was waking up in Mike's bed in a puddle of sweat, or at least that's what I thought it was. I uncovered my head with the stained sheets and noticed Mike staring at me, like a deer in headlights. He was accompanied by a lanky European girl who barely spoke any English. She was wearing a hideous, navy blue romper that was very unflattering. She gave me the death stare and gave Mike the side-eye. She couldn't comprehend why Mike would invite her back to the house when he already had a bun in the oven. I was a soiled bun in the oven so I couldn't imagine that I was very appetizing to Mike. Regardless, I pretended to play it cool while Mike politely pawned the girl in the romper off to one of his roommates. I spent the entire night trying hard to remember how I had gotten in his bed in the first place.

When the show finally aired, I would watch the events unfold like a bad horror movie. Apparently, I had stumbled over to the cast's apartment and stood outside yelling up to the window. Snooki was the only cast member home. She opted out of clubbing for the night to stay home and talk on the phone with her boyfriend, Jionni. Well, she heard me yelling from down below and reluctantly let me in. She could most likely tell that I was wasted; I was tripping over my own wedges and my skirt kept scrunching up, exposing my butt cheeks. She thought it would be funny to "plant" me in Mike's bed so that when he came home with a girl, he would be confronted with a really awkward situation. The plan actually backfired on Snooki, the prankster. When Mike discovered me in his bed, he was relieved. He referred to me as "a bun in the oven." I was already "warmed up," which meant we were one step closer to hooking up. I was already half naked. This equated to less work for him.

We relocated to the Smoosh Room, where we hooked up. We didn't go all the way, thank god. He actually refused, stating that he wasn't ready. I have no idea what that meant but I was more than thrilled with the plan to stay at third base. Watching my actions on TV was borderline traumatic. I also didn't know if I had peed in his bed because all I remember was waking up in a puddle, which I assumed was sweat. I was scared shitless. Was I going to be known as the girl who pissed in the Situation's bed? Now, that would have been a situation concocted for trashy reality television. I could already picture being the laughingstock of the entire show. I would be the laughingstock of the entire world. Fortunately, I didn't pee in the bed. Or, if I did, producers chose not to air it.

Reality TV is an industry that profits from the drunk mishaps of the young generation. From the *Housewives* franchise to *Ex on The Beach*, these shows rely on alcohol to generate fierce drama and unsightly quarrels. These famous drunk TV moments are a disgrace to mankind. It's like a dumpster fire; you can't take your eyes off the drama. The degradation that transpires on these shows should be banned. It's a phenomenon that affects primarily women.

Just take a look at a majority of those TV shows—*The Real Housewives, The Bad Girl's Club, The Real World,* etc. All of these trashy shows feature women getting drunk and arguing with each other. Women have also been labeled "sluts" and "whores" for one-night stands and exhibiting provocative behavior. On the other hand, the men get off scot-free. The women become infamous for their provocative behavior while the men become famous for being a "ladies' man." It's a twisted yet very real spectacle. I witnessed this reality firsthand. I was a spectacle. I was painstakingly pigeon-holed as a wasted white girl. I was branded as a slut and there was nothing I could do about it. I was chump.

CHAPTER 5

Bachelor Pad Blackout

My sister and I failed rule number one: Never participate on reality TV if you're an alcoholic. Instead of dishonorably discharging ourselves from the reality TV platform, we kept pursuing it. We were so humiliated from our *Jersey Shore* stint that we sought a comeback. I didn't want to be remembered as the Situation's hookup. We were both hungry for a second chance. We were thirsty for a resurrection. We were also fame whores. We obsessed over the attention that we received—the lights, the camera, and the infamy.

My sister was in an eating disorder treatment facility, for a third time, when I started applying for shows. Most networks were seeking solely new talent. In other words, they didn't want to cast individuals who had been on TV before. The producers sought fresh faces. This was a massive setback. Not only were we on TV just a few months earlier, but there were two of us. One person is forgettable. But an identical duo is unforgettable. Many people recognized us from *Jersey Shore* because we were the unmistakable twins who hooked up with half the cast.

My sister and I were relentless. We kept pedaling despite obvious impediments. We eventually made the executive decision to hide our past from demanding producers. This was a long shot, but it paid off in the end. We were in contact with a *Bachelor* producer who was casting for a show called *Bachelor Pad*. It was a gameshow spinoff of *The Bachelor* on ABC. The two previous seasons of *Bachelor Pad* starred only past contestants from *The Bachelor* and *The Bachelorette*.

This year, producers threw a curveball into season three. They were scouting fans of the show to participate in the show alongside the veterans. We breezed through the first few video questionnaires and it was time for our in-person interviews, located in Los Angeles.

My sister and I were stoked. We had never been so enthusiastic in our lives. We were working out every day, eating healthy, and practicing our poise. This was our moment to shine. This was our break to detach from the *Jersey Shore* stigma. Our slate wasn't blank, but we were receiving an opportunity to rewrite it.

Producers consistently asked the question, "Have you been on TV before?" My sister and I stuck to our guns and persistently lied. We felt like this was our only chance to slip through the cracks, and that's exactly what happened.

During the sequence of interviews in Los Angeles, we met with a private investigator. He asked us questions regarding any arrests, criminal charges, marriages, and past TV involvement. He poked and prodded. My sister and I supplied the man with two consistent stories and one enormous lie. All the guy had to do was Google our names. He would have come across two gnarly mugshots and 1,001 photos of us alongside, and on top of, the cast of *Jersey Shore*. This alleged private investigator must have never Googled our names, because we got the call two weeks later that we were cast on the show.

This was massive news for two small-town girls from Central Florida. We felt redeemed and restored. We envisioned our execution and delivery on the show. We were sarcastic, witty, and unique. We knew America would fall in love with our goofy personalities. We remained confident, yet humble.

When we arrived in Los Angeles for filming, we were confined to a hotel for three days before the production launched. My sister and I were separated. I can vouch for my sister on this; it was three days of sheer angst and torture. Every scenario invaded my headspace. I asked myself, "Were the other contestants going to be mean like *Jersey Shore*?" "Would we be liked?" "Would I drink too much?" "Would we be voted off the first night?" This movie reel of horrific clips kept spinning in my head.

We were also arriving with a key disadvantage. We were the rookies, the fans who had never set foot in the Bachelor Mansion. The other contestants were familiar with each other. They were also familiar with production, filming, and logistics. We were coming into this debauchery blind as bats. I had no idea that I was going to turn to alcohol as a means of coping. I convinced myself that I would limit my alcohol consumption. This was before I realized that I was a full-fledged alcoholic. I was still very much in denial.

It was the night before the show was going to start filming. I was lounging in my hotel room watching Judge Judy and gorging on a fruit platter from the room service menu. I had also ordered a fillet of fish and some steamed vegetable. It was my attempt at watching my weight. I was one day away from wearing a swimsuit on national TV. I couldn't mess around with the food that I actually wanted—burgers, fries, fried calamari, chicken wings, etc.

I heard a knock at the door and it was a producer with a walkie-talkie in her hand and an earpiece. There were dozens of producers in and out of my room hyping me up for the upcoming production. On this evening, she directed me to a conference room to complete at least an hour of interviewing. These interviews made me nervous. I started sweating and second-guessing myself. When I sat down in the hot seat, I could feel my heart fluttering. I got pins and needles under my armpits and I knew that I had forgotten to put deodorant on. I was breaking out in a sweat and there was nothing I could do about it.

When I scanned the room, I noticed fake plants placed awkwardly around the furniture, producers lining every wall, and a full stash of alcohol lingering near the sink. I jokingly stated, "I need some of that." But it wasn't a joke. I was dead serious. I didn't just *want* a drink; I *needed* one. Without hesitation, a producer wearing a lime green beanie shuffled over to the treasure and poured me a glass of white wine, filled to the brim.

Over the past few weeks of communicating with these people, I knew their methods of operation. Alcohol was conveniently gracing every interview room and photo shoot. It was strategically placed within eyesight. It sat there, waiting for a nervous contestant to require medication. I needed a dose in order to reach my full potential. I was stagnant, reserved, and dry while sober. I couldn't expose these qualities to the world.

I was two overfilled glasses of chardonnay in and I was feeling slightly lightheaded. My voice had risen two decibels and the pitch was annoyingly high. I was talking a mile a minute and trying way too hard to make the producers laugh. I could tell they were getting irritated by my excessive drinking. They probably had ten other contestants to interview that night and they were painstakingly wasting their precious time recording my ranting banter that was most likely unusable material. An hour in, and I saw the woman with the beanie say, "Cut." She did the hand motion and all. She recommended that we resume the interview in the morning when I was a little more "refreshed." I was disappointed. Not in myself, but in the fact that I would have to start drinking early the following morning. Perhaps I would stick to champagne. Maybe make a cute mimosa. I polished off the last bit of wine and lollygagged back to my room.

When I got back, I tore off my clothes and replaced them with comfy pajamas. I swung open the mini fridge and pounded an airplane bottle of Grey Goose. I flew into my bed clutching a room service menu. I said, "Screw it," and ordered a bacon cheeseburger, medium rare. I tuned into the Food Network and waited for my two thousand calories to appear in my lap. I was in heaven. I was in an alcohol-fueled daze. I couldn't be happier. I felt high as a kite.

The last happy memory that I had of the entire experience was in the limo as we pulled up to the mansion and saw Chris Harrison standing in front of the iconic water fountain. This was the very last optimistic thought that would cross my sister's mind and mine before we were thrown into the shit storm. Despite previously being on reality TV, we were unprepared for this storm. We were two amateur storm watchers, riding out a category 5 hurricane in a hut constructed from sticks and hay. We were hours away from being blown away into the night. Our reputations and our self-worth were at stake. Regardless, we took our chances and stepped out of that limo to greet Chris Harrison.

The moment I walked through the doors of the Mansion, I was overwhelmed with anxiety. I immediately regretted my reckless decision. My introversion creeped in and I became reluctant, fearful, and nervous. Everyone appeared so comfortable around each other. I felt like the fat kid in elementary school. I felt like an outcast; I felt inferior. The contestants were flirtatious, boisterous, and catty. They were gregarious and fearless. They spoke their minds and weren't afraid of the cameras—at least they appeared that way. They hated my sister and me. They called us "annoying and immature." You are supposed to have thick skin for reality TV, but my sister and I did not. Our skin was thinner than cheap toilet paper. The comments hurt. They stung deep. They stirred up my feelings of inadequacy and disgrace.

Speaking of grace, alcohol was my saving grace. The moment I started drinking, I felt fearless. I returned at least eight times to the bar to refill my drink on that first night. I needed that liquid courage and I know my sister felt the same way. The bar was an alcoholic's dream come true. There was every conceivable brand and flavor of liquor. Everything was top-shelf and all the bottles were full. My heart sang. This was my lifeline and my worst enemy.

The moment we stepped foot in the mansion, my sister and I practiced social isolation, and not because the coronavirus was going around. We were tense and petrified. We were not social butterflies by nature. We clung together, like Siamese twins. This is a common habit among twins. We clung to each other in times of distress. Even with the consumption of booze, we were scared shitless.

We survived night one without completely humiliating ourselves. We were the last contestants to arrive at the party and, therefore, started drinking later than everyone else. This circumstance saved us. There was no doubt that we would have blacked out if we had arrived any earlier. God was on our side.

The next day I woke up feeling refreshed and relatively sober. This was an extraordinary feat in my repertoire of boozing. We sensed that the other contestants were frustrated with the presence of fans in the mansion because we hadn't earned our spot on *Bachelor Pad.* Apparently, we hadn't "got dumped on national TV." They had no idea that we had, in fact, been humiliated on national TV, just not dumped by the bachelor.

On the first day, we were given a challenge that would give the winning couple immunity from elimination and the losing couple a vote against them. When we walked outside of the mansion into the front terrace, we were greeted by seven giant hearts, made of wood. These contraptions were large enough to fit two people inside of them and were suspended into the air. We had to wedge ourselves into the heart-shaped box and basically hang without falling out. Whoever stayed in the heart-shaped boxes the longest were the winners. This was literally the easiest thing I've ever had to do in my life. I could have sat, wedged in that heart all day. The other contestants were sweating and groaning. They were dropping like flies. Within ten minutes, I was the last man hanging.

When my sister and I won the first challenge, we received even more adverse feedback because we were safe from going home. The entire house had planned on voting us out first. By winning, we were unknowingly throwing a wrench in the other contestants' unanimous plan. I felt alone, shunned, and miserable. All I wanted to do was drink and forget where I was.

Since we won the challenge, we were rewarded with a date night at the Santa Monica Pier with our male partner on the show. During the date, we had a glass of alcohol in our hands at all times; I couldn't function with it and I certainly couldn't function without it. We drank throughout the entire night—I couldn't stop. I needed it for clarity, and I needed it for my anxiety. The last thing I remember is my sister passed out. She was lying sprawled across the center row of the white production van. Producers were insistently handing her bottles of water to sober her up. She was gone. I was shortly behind her.

When I woke up the next morning, my head was screaming for more booze. My brain was murky and my body was frail. I could barely wobble down the stairs without losing my balance. My withdrawals, disguised as hangovers, were my little secret. I didn't want the world to witness my withdrawals; they certainly weren't for the faint of heart. My symptoms were ugly and distasteful, nothing that my fellow castmates could relate to. I felt even more alone.

I causally scrolled downstairs around 10 a.m. and started concocting a Bloody Mary because that's what contestants on reality TV do, right? With a camera in my face, recording my every move, I chugged the vodka with tomato juice. I immediately felt more amicable; I could function again. Most importantly, I could complete my confessional interviews without feeling nauseous and shaky.

By nightfall, my sister and I were shitfaced, for lack of a better adjective. I was blacked out by noon and I don't remember a damn thing. I vaguely remember arguing with my sister. I think she called me a whore. We went at it like we were starring on an episode of *Jerry Springer*. We carried ourselves like white trash. We were slurring our words and behaving like juveniles. Every single contestant loathed our high-pitched voices. We were two animals that needed to be exterminated. I was barely able to stand during the first rose ceremony. If we didn't hold immunity from winning the first challenge, we would have been eliminated, right then and there. I was supposed to hand out the roses during the ceremony, but I was too intoxicated.

By sunrise, my sister and I had packed up our belongings and left the show. I was angry at myself for drinking like a fool. I was angry at myself for exposing my alcoholism, which I couldn't even control for one week. It reared its ugly head during my most vulnerable times. That's the thing about addiction; you can't control it under any circumstance.

When the show aired, I was mortified. It was almost worse than our *Jersey Shore* charade. Watching yourself on the big screen in a total blackout is excruciating. I don't wish it upon my worst enemy. I looked into my own eyes, on that screen, and witnessed a girl possessed by alcohol. My actions and behaviors were infantile and humiliating. I refused to believe that I was watching myself. I was intelligent, witty, and beautiful; I was not that hideous and repulsive contestant on *Bachelor Pad*.

This was our only chance to restore our reputation and we unequivocally blew it faster and harder than an air horn. The reality TV scene is simply not cut out for an alcoholic. It's an environment that oozes alcohol. The temptation to continuously drink is prevalent and profound. It was an alcoholic booby trap. I didn't learn my lesson the first go-around, and I repeated history. I hated myself. Most importantly, I hated my alcoholism.

I had always dreamed of being famous. The infamy that my sister and I had built was a nightmare. Our TV experiences had ignited a dangerous fire. Strangers trolled the internet for opportunities to spew hate. On camera, our fellow contestants expressed their disdain for my sister and me. We were annoying, yappy dogs that belonged on a show like *Maury*. I didn't disagree with this evaluation. What I didn't appreciate were strangers putting their two cents in where it didn't belong. These "haters" were awful and relentless. If I were suicidal, I would have pulled the trigger. Strangers called us "sluts," "fame whores," "ugly," and "nasty." To the online world, we were a disgrace. In Gainesville, we were local celebrities.

Jersey Shore was the number one show among college students. Almost every individual within the demographic tuned into *Jerzday*. We were recognized in class, at the bar, and even in the gym. We couldn't go anywhere without a stranger requesting a picture. I went from partying every weekend to partying every night. I craved the attention just as much as I craved alcohol.

Every night, my sister and I coordinated our outfits, banged a few shots, and hit the bars. We were a dynamic duo. We felt popular and prevalent. It was a six-month period of my life that was thrilling and chaotic. I was wholly out of my element and certainly not accustomed to the attention that we received. Fortunately, alcohol was a major piece of the pie. It was our rock through every rough patch. We drank to manipulate our thoughts and actions.

I joke that I had to be wasted when I watched *Jersey Shore* for the first time. Unaware of what MTV would air, I needed a potential emotional eraser. I had blacked out four out of the five nights that I was "stalking" the cast and did not trust my drunk persona. She was a tornado—unpredictable and treacherous. Her provocative spirit was a monster that I didn't want exposed to the world.

Watching myself on TV wasn't half bad while half in the bag. My behavior appeared less appalling and my actions were less outrageous. I had to rewatch the "Twinning" episode because I drank four shots too many during the pregame. I didn't remember a damn thing. Blacking out was the easiest way to cope with a worst-case scenario. It was my go-to.

CHAPTER 6

New York City of Dreams

I was done with reality TV and I was done with college. I had extended my stay. The party scene was no longer giving me that high that it used to. I had always dreamed of moving to New York City and building a life as a New Yorker. I had it stipulated in my head how my dream would play out. I would find an older, wealthy man to marry. We would have three kids, live in a colossal penthouse in Manhattan, and drive BMWs. I would lunch with my high-profile counterparts and attend charity events on my wealthy husband's arm. I would sip expensive champagne and mingle with influential, beautiful people. Everyone would be envious of my life.

The adverse attention that I received in college would become a distant cry. I was going to reemerge as a new woman. This woman would embody respect, success, and clout. I would turn over a new leaf; this was my metamorphosis from a girl to a woman.

I have always been under the impression that pretty people get things in life. They have the capability to obtain whatever they want simply because of their appearance. I will confess, I thought I was a pretty girl. I knew I wasn't beautiful, but my personality would make up for those shortcomings. I truly believed that I could become *someone* simply by meeting the right man and climbing the social ladder via the right people. The delusion that I faced during this time in my life was insidious.

I had grown up with a mother who modeled hard work and dedication. How and when did my delusional mentality materialize? The answer to that question is simple. I drowned myself in alcohol throughout my four years in college, which completely took a toll on my brain. My thought processes and patterns were stunted to the point where I became delusional and pretentious. That's what alcohol does. It fries your insides. It hijacks your brain into seeing the world through the eyes of a drunk. Your dreams and aspirations become after-thoughts in a mind that prioritizes partying. Alcohol slowly and meticulously drains you of stamina and tenacity.

Alcohol doesn't want you to succeed. It's selfish. It demands your attention by forcing you to neglect all other prerogatives. Other obligations fall to the wayside in a deliberate and progressive cycle. Before you know it, typical college partying devolves into alcohol abuse. Once you reach this category, it's only a matter of time until you admit that you're an alcoholic. That's a scary word, even to an alcoholic.

My move to New York was a slapdash endeavor. It was a poorly thought-out arrangement that left me in a precarious predicament. I was scrolling through Craigslist looking for someone who was exchanging room and board for house cleaning and dog walking. Yes, you read that correctly. I was seeking a free place to stay, expecting to clean that individual's house daily in return. I was deranged. Despite common sensibility, I proceeded with an arrangement to move to Flushing, Queens.

I remember browsing Craigslist while I was at work as a bartender in Gainesville. I was working at a dive bar that smelled like a bowling alley. It reeked of burnt grease and carpet that was saturated with cheap beer. It was a Monday and I probably had about two people sit at the bar. My phone was glued to my hand; I was determined to secure a place to stay in New York. Most ads that I stumbled upon were sketchy. I could tell that most of the men were seeking some type of sexual arrangement in exchange for room and board. I investigated and analyzed every post, trying to identify the serial killers. After much deliberation, I kept being drawn back to this man who had a three-bedroom apartment in Queens. I spoke to him on the phone three times before I proceeded with the move. He alleged that I would have the entire upper floor to myself. Once he made the remark that he had a girlfriend, I was sold. Because murderers and rapists don't have girlfriends. Instead, they reel you in under false pretenses in a creepy, predictable manner. I had saved up $200, packed two suitcases, and was off to the Big Apple.

When I arrived in New York, I had zero expectations. Well, I had one expectation: not to be murdered. I climbed in a rinky-dink yellow cab at JFK Airport. I remember a gust of frosty air sending chills down my spine. For a split second, I second-guessed my decision to move from paradise to the arctic. I couldn't go back now; there were no refunds. I used my mom's Discover card to pay for the ride because I only had the $200 and I had already spent $20 of it binging on Wendy's at the Orlando Airport. My mom insisted that I use her credit card in emergencies. I deemed this an emergency.

The cab pulled up in front of a dingy ramshackle. If I didn't know any better, I would have thought we were in Chinatown on Canal Street. Every single person was Asian. My new roommate and I were the exception. We stuck out like a sore thumb.

Over time, I would begin to embrace the ethnic makeup of my new neighborhood. I would spend the tail end of the night walking home from the subway station that was approximately two miles away from my new house. I grew increasingly comfortable with the neighborhood; no one troubled or harassed me. I never once heard a catcall or a whistle from an unsuspecting onlooker. The Asians were very reclusive, soft-spoken, and restrained. They were private people.

As I jumped out of the cab, a man with bloodshot eyes and a cigarette hanging out of his mouth met me at the door. He nervously chuckled and commented on my bright, summery clothes with open-toed shoes. He seemed a little "out of it." I could tell he was nervous, which appeased my anxiety. He grabbed the broken handle to my suitcase and we walked up the seedy flight of stairs. I couldn't help but notice a thick layer of dust and dog hair caked to the floorboards and the railings. The apartment reeked of pot and cigarette smoke accompanied by a paralyzing aroma of spicy Persian food. I could smell the turmeric and the saffron smothering whatever meat he was roasting.

The man seemed decent, yet too high on marijuana to function. He spoke in a dialect that resembled a mix of English, Hebrew, and stoner. He proceeded to roll a fat doobie and advised me to get comfortable upstairs, where I would be staying. The man seemed harmless. After partaking in some light banter, he stated, "I'm so relieved that you're not some psycho bitch." We actually hit it off really well. We possessed the same sense of dark humor and laid-back demeanor. I could tell that his brain was fried. He was too shot to execute anything dangerous. If he did murder me, he would be too stoned to dispose of my body. He would be screwed.

I was sitting on the mushy leather couch when my mind started churning. The man, named Avi, hadn't yet given me a tour of our abode. I had no idea where I would be resting my head at night. I envisioned a dainty, adorable room with a floral bedspread and clean towels neatly folded on the edge of the bed. I fantasized about the quaint bathroom stocked with feminine necessities—shaving cream, conditioner, and perhaps Summer's Eve. The large window would be draped with classic, outdated curtains, and the pastel carpet would be slightly frayed from the minimal amount of foot traffic. This was not the case.

As I walked up the second flight of stairs to reach my personal dwelling, I became nauseated. The smell of stale dog poop and stagnant, musty cigarette smoke overwhelmed my senses. As I stood at the top of the stairs, I looked to the left. I saw a microscopic room stuffed with gigantic drums and musical equipment. The floor was littered with large mounds of dried dog poop, a total of three landmines. The repugnant smell of dog urine lurked in the room. I wanted to vomit.

Perhaps my room would be more presentable. I pivoted to my right and took four baby steps toward my room. I noticed the cheap carpet was blanketed with dirt; I couldn't even decipher the original color. The doorway had nails protruding from the floorboard as if the carpet was being ripped out. The room was missing a door. That was a relief. If I was moving in with a psycho serial killer, it would certainly be the opposite. There would be a fortification of doors with intricate locks to ensure the maintenance of his victims. This was assuredly not the workings of a deranged serial kidnapper. It was the disarray and wreckage of a man who was too addicted to marijuana to care about the aesthetics of his anarchic abode.

This was going to be an impeccable match. Two addicts, two different drugs of choice, two people who gave zero fucks—and most prominently, we were two people who derived happiness from a substance. As long as we had alcohol and weed, we were golden. We would be happier than flies on shit.

My room was meager and limited. There was a full-sized blow-up mattress underneath the modest, hazy window. The room was blotched with patches of dirty carpet. Underneath was antiquated, dark wood floors from the mid-1900s that were speckled with white paint. The bathroom was cramped and desolate. There was no shower curtain, and when I flipped the light, a loud popping noise almost blew out my eardrum. The socket must have shorted because when I gave the light another whirl, nothing happened. I didn't care. I was content with my space. It was shoddy and subpar, but it was mine. I think I was just relieved that I was still alive and not murdered shortly after my arrival.

By evening, I had the entire apartment cleaned to a tee. I bleached every tile, scrubbed every inch, and vacuumed every crumb. My new roommate was utterly impressed. He was grateful that I wasn't some heroin addict looking to pawn his personal items.

That very first night, my roommate invited me out with his friend to a bar in the city. I contemplated whether I should go or not. I had made a vow to myself that I wouldn't party half as much as I did in college. I was here to work and find my future husband. There would be no more stints in the hospital from alcohol poisoning, no more random hookups and STDs, and certainly no more arrests for disorderly conduct. My new life in New York would be responsible, respectable, and of course rewarding.

Despite my gut telling me to stay home, I wanted to bond with my new roommate. I was fearful that my drunken alter ego would send my new roomie running for the hills. Blacking out was a regular occurrence in my repertoire of binges. I rolled the dice every single time I took that first sip of alcohol. On that evening, I would become a slave to Grey Goose.

My roomie and I shared a couple drinks and we headed out into the city via the seven train. I remember sitting on the cold, hard subway seat ruminating about my future. I was not only physically inebriated; I was mentally intoxicated as well. That subway ride confirmed my arrival in the city of dreams. It was a testimony to my journey. I had made it to the Big Apple, with $180 in my pocket and a backpack full of dreams and delusions.

When we stepped off the subway platform, all the blood rushed to my head. I was in a daze, but I pulled it together for the sake of my new relationship with a stranger. We arrived at his friend's glossy, high-rise apartment on 80th Street on the Upper East Side. The elevator ride to the 23rd floor seemed eternal. I was already yearning for more alcohol. I needed it to ease my anxiety. I needed copious amounts of alcohol to break out of my introverted shell, which I detested. Alcohol was my survival guide and my only tool. It was my only means to acquiring the fearlessness that was mandatory in every free-spirited endeavor that I embarked on.

Let's face it, sober individuals make rational, lucid, and impartial decisions in relation to their lives. My actions and behaviors were reckless, audacious, and poorly constructed. The term "free spirit" is a euphemism for acting young and stupid.

As I sat on the plush white couch of this stranger's apartment, I became entranced. I sipped my Grey Goose martini like a class act. The apartment was polished, modern, and chic. It was a bachelor pad on steroids. I scrutinized the oversized abstract artwork on the wall. The colors were intoxicating. The glass-blown figurines that delicately adorned the space coordinated with the wall art. The marble and granite countertops in the kitchen were graced with fragile framed pictures. I speculated that the man's girlfriend had a hand in the interior design. I surmised that she was an executive assistant for some fashion designer on Fifth Avenue. She was polished, beautiful, and classy. This fictitious girlfriend embodied every quality and style that I sought.

When I snapped back into reality, I craved another drink. Perhaps, if I drank myself into oblivion, I could assume the form of this mystery girlfriend and achieve her status.

Drinking is magical. Its ability to transcend my consciousness into a fantastical dimension was enchanting. It took me out of reality for a night. It eradicated my self-doubt and gave me confidence that all of my whims could become reality.

My roommate motioned me to join him outside on the balcony. I stood and gathered my balance to disguise my intoxication. I walked out onto the balcony and a rush of cold, raw, winter air smacked me in the face. My roomie handed me a fat, hand-rolled joint and I warily took a healthy drag. I was instantaneously removed from reality at that point. The last thing I remembered from that night was fumbling in my purse for my ID at the front door of a strip club. I vaguely recall ordering a vodka and Diet Coke from the bar and the rest was history. Another blackout was added to my repository of forgotten, drunken nights.

I woke up the next morning on a flattened, deflated air mattress in my new chamber. I was alleviated when I became cognizant of the fact that I didn't wake up in someone else's bed, particularly my new roommate's. Well, that was a first. Had I turned a corner? I was proud of this magnanimous modification in my previous whorish behavior. I felt classy.

For twenty years, I was entangled in a chase. I was invariably chasing things that I understood would irrevocably make me happy. I speculated that moving to New York would satisfy my yearning for the big city. I chased money, inferring that it was the root of all my problems. I chased love, concluding that it was the missing element in my life. I chased the highs of drinking and I chased the highs of sex. After acquiring all these ingredients, I was still miserable.

The conundrum of life's infinite quest for happiness is simply an illusion. We assume that we must embark on life's endeavors to achieve and acquire things; once fulfilled, happiness will prevail. This is simply a bogus story that we tell ourselves throughout life. Why not be happy today regardless of where we are and what we have?

CHAPTER 7

M is for Men with Money

Two days into my pilgrimage, I landed a job as a cocktail waitress at an upscale cigar bar on the Upper East Side. The establishment itself was a poorly lit lair underneath a southern BBQ restaurant on 68th Street and First Avenue. Accepting that job at Merchant's Cigar Bar would fundamentally be the most pivotal life decision among all of the poor and shortsighted choices I would make over the ensuing four years. Merchant's would become the backdrop for all of my devious and forbidden behavior. I was an alcoholic working at a bar; I was a monkey selling bananas and I was elated. I was proud because I was employed.

This dingy cigar bar fascinated me. It was the watering well for many successful Wall Streeters, hedge fund owners, celebrities, and rappers. The clientele essentially encompassed a slew of older, wealthy men, willing and able to spend their hard-earned money. This was *my* watering hole. This was my hunting ground. The second a man walked through the stairwell, I was analyzing and executing my attack. I stalked my prey and marked bull's-eyes on my budding victims. I audited and inspected each patron the moment he stepped foot into my establishment. I scrutinized his appearance for any cracks, any sign that he was not wealthy. I scanned his buttoned-up shirt for fresh iron marks and made sure his shoes were polished and untarnished. I scanned his wrists for expensive, gaudy watches. Lastly, I scanned his ring fingers for any sign of commitment. A wedding ring was in no way a deterrent; in fact, it was a preference of mine. The married men were easier to deal with. They were discreet, undemanding, and uncomplicated. They expected nothing but sex. They were simple transactions that never required a receipt.

My commute into the city was daunting to say the least. The exact distance from work to home was ten miles but it seemed like a world away. Avi's apartment to the subway station was exactly one and a half miles from the Main Street subway station. It was the very last stop on the seven train. Once I got to the station by foot, I was already exhausted. The station itself was an ant farm. It was overcrowded with Asians practically bumping into each other. It smelled like pork fried rice and hot, steamy garbage. Once I boarded the train, I was just one sardine amongst hundreds. The Asians never offered me their seat; I usually stood all the way to the Lexington stop.

Standing during a subway ride was not my strong suit. Every time the train jerked, I was falling into someone or stepping on toes. I was a mess. I popped my earbuds into my ears and listened to Taylor Swift and One Direction. I was the whitest girl on the train. When I arrived at the station, I transferred to the six train, which then went uptown for a few stops. Walking up the stairs of the 62nd station was cathartic. I felt like I had just run a half marathon. I felt dirty yet thankful that I had arrived.

The Upper East Side was my turf. I was in love with the tree-lined streets, posh boutique shops, and cute little cafes. I yearned to live there. I hoped that one day I would be *that* mom, pushing a $500 stroller with $5 coffee in her hand. Every woman who lived on the Upper East Side wore overpriced spandex with matching Nikes. They probably didn't even work out. They just looked cute. I didn't want to bartend, and I certainly didn't want to be a cocktail server. I wanted to be financially free. I wanted to be a stay-at-home mom.

It took about two weeks to acclimate to the cigar culture and environment. I felt compelled to practice sobriety in these weeks of transition as I cultivated the knowledge of cigars, aged scotches, and fine wines. Keep in mind, I had been a bartender at a dive bar back in Gainesville, Florida. My most demanding challenge was learning the dance moves to the "Wobble," which we'd performed on the bar during games. I was charting new territory: I was working at a formal and refined establishment that required knowledge, charm, and professionalism from their cocktail servers. I was a chameleon. I had every single owner, manager, and coworker fooled into believing my top-notch waitressing finesse and expertise. I helped my coworkers in every way that I could. I covered shifts for girls who were sick and even turned down the conventional after-work drinks with my coworkers. I was sober, attentive, and eager.

Six weeks into my new endeavor, I became reasonably comfortable and complacent. My cocktail dresses got progressively shorter and my stilettos got significantly higher. I initiated flirtatious banter with my prospects and cautiously played my cards with the hand that I was dealt. It's much smoother to play your cards in a sober state of mind. Once I cracked open that first beer, I was showing players my cards, folding with royal flushes, and betting all my chips with a pair of deuces. Regardless of these crippling odds, I rolled the dice.

Three months after moving to Queens, the relationship with Avi started to crumble. We were like newlyweds who married in Vegas after knowing each other for eight weeks. He established basic rules and I broke every single one of them. He was becoming frustrated with my mischiefs. One night, I invited this guy back to our place. I was intoxicated and barely remembered the night. My date and I were fooling around on the couch when I heard Avi climbing the stairs. I felt like I was in high school and my parents just walked in on me kissing a boy. I was too drunk to care. I repeatedly apologized as the man slinked out of the apartment with his tail between his legs. He never brought up the incident, but I could tell he was pissed.

He was smoking more weed than usual, and I was sneaking vodka from his giant bottle of Grey Goose. Despite the failing arrangement, I knew I had to move closer to my job. It was too risky taking the subway at four in the morning, drunk and stumbling. I needed to accommodate my alcoholism, so I rented a makeshift room from a creepy little Argentinian man, two blocks away from the cigar bar. The man's apartment was originally built as a studio. He constructed a wall smack dab in the middle of the room, creating a tiny space that I would inhabit for the ensuing three months.

I caved in and began regularly participating in shenanigans with coworkers. I even locked lips with my manager so that he would favor me over the other servers. Drinking at the dive bar across the street after work gradually turned into having a few shots at work with my patrons. Naturally, having a few drinks at work *with* the regulars turned into bringing a small bottle of vodka to work every single night.

It wasn't long before I could hardly endure a full eight-hour shift without drinking. Drinking eased my mind and warmed my personality. With a couple of swigs, I morphed into a charismatic, gregarious, and almost fatuous girl that men seemed to gravitate toward. I had gained a few pounds since my move to the city and I had temporarily extinguished my eating disorder for the time being. Alcohol made me feel sexy, skinny, carefree, and confident. It was medicine for my insecurity.

I was getting ready for work on a frigid November night. Now that I was stationed a few blocks from work, I was happy. No more long commutes back to Queens in zero-degree weather wearing shitty, off-brand Ugg boots that were sopping with melted snow. I was officially an Upper East Sider.

As I caked layers and layers of mascara on my eyelashes and drew thick black eyeliner underneath my eyes, I swigged from a warm bottle of Skinny Girl Margarita that probably should have been refrigerated. This gave me the energy and anticipation that I needed to endure an entire night shift.

When I finally got to work, I jumped into the grind. I set the candles on the tables, prepared the cigar boxes, and wiped down the menus. Patrons began trickling in and I was getting increasingly irritable. I was highly unhappy with the rotation of tables; every table of mine was demeaning and cheap as fuck. I needed more alcohol. My tank was low, and I was running on fumes. My gas light had turned on an hour ago and I was penetrating desperation. I couldn't fake one more smile nor fabricate another cheesy, superficial conversation.

The night finally hit a lull around nine; I darted out the door and beelined to the neighboring liquor store. I was still wearing five-inch heels and I could feel the cold overwhelm my pudgy body. My toes were frozen and my lips were blue. I asked the clerk for a pint of Smirnoff, minus the paper bag. I hated that little paper bag. It was just a paper trail. It was evidence for any suspecting outsider looking in; the only people who buy vodka by the pint are alcoholics. Every alcoholic can relate to the irritation precipitated from that little bag. What is it for? It literally only hides the label, but it doesn't take a shitty psychic to reveal the contents.

I returned to work and scampered to the coatroom, where I had secured my personal items. I took three gulps of the hundred-proof Smirnoff. My throat burned with excitement. I made this "ahh" sound as if I had just taken a sip of an ice-cold Coca-Cola. This was not Coca-Cola. This was medicinal poison.

I strutted out of that coat closet with a newfound certainty and clarity. I felt revitalized. I sparked up arbitrary conversations with strangers and even dropped drinks off at tables that weren't mine. I bobbed my head back and forth and swung my hair to the rhythm of the drowned-out music. I was in Brittany Land. Brittany Land was a sweet and luscious place, like Candy Land. It was a mental space that encircled every fantastical quality of reality. It was joyous, provocative, and self-indulgent. In Brittany Land, everyone adores and envies me. It's an egotistical headspace that gives me an undeniable sense of assurance and enchantment. It was called being drunk.

It was approximately 10:20 p.m. when I saw the shadow of a man walk into the bar. As I approached him, the first thing I noticed was his thick, black-rimmed glasses complemented by his disheveled, thick black hair. He had white earbuds in his ears and a slouchy briefcase draped over his slouchy shoulders. He was mysterious. His white buttoned-up shirt was neatly ironed and unblemished, at first glance. You could see the wear-and-tear of a tumultuous day written all over his wrinkled face. He hastily snagged a table, and another cocktail server scrambled to his side before I even had an opportunity to explore this man even more.

As I walked back and forth between tables, I caught the man glaring at me. He was fixated and I was intrigued. Why were my coworkers so adamant on acquiring this table, which consisted of one paltry person? Was he some celebrity or simply a wealthy man who tipped hundreds of dollars?

The manager of the bar informed me that this man, Brooks, tipped hundreds of dollars on tabs that maxed out at $50. He proceeded to tell me that Brooks had requested my service. What? Why? Me? This Merchant's celebrity and benefactor wants *me* to serve him?

I felt honored and overwhelmed and zero remorse for my coworker, who thought she was going to score a couple hundred dollars that evening. The pressure to perform was crushing my ego. I needed another drink. What did I need to perform? I wasn't sure. The man definitively had needs. I was apprehensive. How would I "earn" such a robust tip? There must be a catch-22 in this scenario. Men don't just throw money at unsuspecting women and expect nothing in return. I *knew* men.

I was two shots deep in a matter of ten minutes. He had only one Johnnie Walker Black under his belt and I could tell that he was feeling unhinged. He asked me creepy questions regarding the color of my undergarments and the types of things that turn me on. I answered every question based on what I thought the desperate man desired to hear. This pathetic soul sat in a bar, interrogating women for his own sick and twisted gratification. He described his fantasies in detail, including having sex in a bed full of hundred-dollar bills. Assuming that these bills were fresh off the press, of course I loved that fantasy.

This man loved money, scotch, and sex. His family was clearly *not* on his mind. We were two peas in a pod, except for the fact that he was twenty years my senior. He was virtually a senior citizen.

I was enthralled. I needed more of this man. It was a combination of his solitary, nerdy appearance and his cryptic demeanor that kept me yearning for more verbal exchanges. The man got drunk surprisingly quick for a grown, adult man. He got sloppy and reckless. I knew he was married before he even disclosed that arbitrary information. He was a man crying out for attention. His mind was perverted and vast. He appreciated my humble roots. His captivation and obsession with my passion, my energy, and my blonde hair was undeniable.

When he asked for the check at midnight, my heart started fluttering. I couldn't contain my excitement. I had schmoozed and buttered this man up for two protracted hours. I periodically stroked his ego, played into his games, and deliberately turned him on. I felt like he *owed* me.

I hastily swung open the greasy, little black checkbook and my squinty, drunk eyes became wide. Benjamin Franklin stared right back at me. There, in my hands, were six perfectly crisp hundred-dollar bills. This amount of cash jolted my soul. I had just won the lottery. This man was a whale. I was just a tiny fish in this big sea. I desired more and would do anything for it.

As he made his way to the door, he whispered in my ear. I could feel droplets of spit coat my ear canal. He slurred the words "Meet me outside" as he slithered out of the door, like a snake. I ran up the carpeted stairs and halted when I saw Brooks leaning against the hand railing, literally holding himself up from tumbling back into the bar. He drunkenly muttered that he wanted to kiss me. I was high, jubilant, and a willing participant. He proceeded to smother me with his wet, sloppy lips. He was indulgent and careless and lacked delicacy and sensuality. I thought to myself, *It's no wonder his wife won't have sex with this grown man whose behavior was grossly atrocious.* He was a desperate puppy dog pursing a leg to hump. He was a lion in heat. He was an animal. Despite the initial shock of being ravaged by an animal, I was just satisfied and content that it was over.

Brooks went into hibernation for the ensuing two weeks. Maybe he was ashamed, or perhaps mama bear smelled the scent of another animal on his clothes when he returned home the other night. Was he not allowed out? Or was he evading me? My mind exhausted every rationalization.

When Brooks returned to the lair, also known as Merchant's, I was alleviated, and so was my TD Bank account. Depositing cash into my bank account would become my new obsession. I was infatuated with cold, hard cash. I was even more infatuated with the man who provided it. He was my shiny new ATM machine. From that point on, I never used my mom's Discover card ever again.

Brooks seemed soft-pedaled on that night. He was more restrained and composed. I fixed this glitch with a cumbersome pour of Johnnie Walker Black. Brooks instantaneously reappeared to his unrefined and unequivocal self. This night was epic. It was the inauguration of our contorted, bent narrative. Brooks would make modest strides every time we colluded. On that night, he insisted that we have a drink at the bar across the street when my shift was over. The bar was named "Honky Tonk." It was not decent, but it was discreet. It was an establishment that guaranteed Brooks' anonymity. He was not going to run into his wife, his coworkers, or his comrades in this shithole. It was a perfect refuge—his retreat from the woes of married life, and my retreat from the terrible twenties.

We sat in the back room of the bar on a bench that we shared. The bar didn't have Johnnie Walker Black so Brooks begrudgingly drank Johnnie Walker Red. I drank a double of Three Olives, Fruity Loops, with ice. It was essentially vodka that tasted like the Fruit Loops cereal. My choice in drink reminded Brooks of our age disparity. I think he welcomed my childlike, infantile side. Brooks was a child himself. His humor was sophomoric and immature, despite his undeniable intelligence.

For three hours we kissed each other like we were in high school. He aggressively rubbed my thighs up and down like it was his first time touching a female. He slobbered on my neck, jammed his tongue in my mouth, and nibbled on my ear like it was going out of style. I felt violated and impassioned at the same time. His eyes were half-open, and I could tell he was wasted. He kept repeating himself. His compliments were compulsive. "You're so sexy, you're so hot, you're so sexy, you're so hot..." He was a broken record, but I didn't hate it. I felt broken at this point in my life and his affirmations made me feel a little less damaged.

The clock stroked midnight and we were both two sheets to the wind. I proceeded with the customary invitation back to my place. Going back to his place obviously wasn't in the running. I didn't feel like sharing a king-sized bed with his wife. I also wasn't in the appropriate condition to chitchat with his kids. Brooks suggested reluctance when I threw the offer on the table. His wheels were spinning.

I pictured his presumably beautiful wife at home. She would be awaiting his return, draped in an all-white silk robe. She passed the evening hours immersed in a crime fiction novel as she lay on the ottoman that graced the end of their bed. She had just put the four kids to sleep, two girls and two boys. She anticipated her husband while he was simply decompressing with a glass of scotch and a cigar on this innocent Tuesday night. I shortly returned to reality.

Indeed, Brooks was decompressing. He was literally unraveling at the seams. The life that he had built was in fact compressing and very heavy. The burdens of daily life were altering this man's happiness. He was overly involved and drained. He needed to escape, but only for a night. He had way too many obligations and commitments as a husband, a father, and a businessman. He required multiple days of retrieve, but he would settle for a couple hours with me. The next two hours would feel like a lifetime of unraveling. He was about to collapse.

My Upper East Side roommate was a creepy Argentinian man who worked as an architect and drove an old 2001 Porsche. He spent the winters at his home in Costa Rica; therefore, the entire apartment was mine to exploit. We stumbled back to my apartment. With hesitation, I poured us both a shot of cheap vodka. He vetoed my offering because one more drink would incapacitate him. The same rang true for me. Regardless, I downed my shot and his as well. I needed alcohol to participate in the foolishness that would ensue.

The last thing I remembered was flinging the cushions off the couch and rattling open the latent sofa bed. The metal hinges screeched and the aroma of a stale, mildewed mattress filled the room. It was either the sofa bed or the air mattress, and I made the executive decision to go with option A. I woke up the next morning with my head spinning off its axis. The room looked fuzzy, but not as fuzzy as the night before. I grabbed the bottle of Smirnoff next to the bed and guzzled two healthy gulps. My head immediately stopped spinning. I could focus again.

I was feeling nauseous already, but the thought of hooking up with an old man nauseated me even more. My bra was still fastened but my panties were misplaced. I loathed myself in that very moment, as I normally did. What happened last night? Did I bring Brooks home or did we say our farewells at the bar? I vaguely remember his presence inside my pint-sized quarters. If only he would have consumed his shot of vodka instead of me, I wouldn't have blacked out. My alcoholism consisted of boundless what-ifs. I never took full accountability and always attributed my drunken plights to extraneous factors. I blamed Brooks for buying me drinks. I blamed him for trailing me home. And, I blamed him for allowing me to take that last shot.

As I grazed my hand over the bedspread to look for my phone, I noticed it was soiled. The already sour, stagnant mattress just got even more rotten. This poor, dinky mattress had not only witnessed the atrocities of the preceding night but had endured them. I mobilized my thoughts to create an innocent excuse for the sodden sheets. Perhaps, Brooks spilled some water or maybe the ceiling was leaking.

I damn well knew the source of the sop. This was a common reality that plagued me all throughout college. I experienced a surplus of mortifying moments while drunk, most of which I don't remember. Unfortunately, this embarrassing habit didn't tolerate forgetfulness, because I was always reminded when I woke up in a puddle of my own piss. You would think that urinating the bed like a baby would give a person an indication that they have a drinking problem. Googling "Drunk bedwetting" yields results that are somewhat reassuring. Apparently, involuntary urination while intoxicated is a real thing. It's a phenomenon that almost two percent of adults have experienced. Thank you, Google, for convincing me that I'm not an alcoholic.

After a slapdash attempt at partially piecing together my rendezvous with the old, rich guy, I considered shooting him a text. Then I reevaluated; I contemplated that very action. Brooks had made it clear that I couldn't text him.

It was the first indication of what our future relationship would consist of. It wasn't long before he would set absolute, ridged boundaries that I had to adhere to. He was married, he had a life; I would become solely an accessory. He would make the arrangements, set the rules, and inevitably deliver the verdicts. He would be the judge. I would be the defendant. I would zip my mouth and comply. There would be days that I was sentenced to prison. I had to follow a scrupulous order; I would be confined, and I couldn't reach out. Then there would be days that I would be acquitted, free to call and text. Some days I would be paroled; I would retain limited freedom if the underlining rules were withstood. Finally, there was death row: I would pretend like Brooks didn't exist; he would be dead to me.

I waited patiently for his correspondence. I waited two long days. I thought I had scared him away. Perhaps I had peed directly on him—I wasn't sure. My thoughts nearly dismantled me. I thought I had ruined my chances with Brooks. He was the man I had always dreamed of. He was a wealthy, quirky, dark-haired Jewish man. Most importantly, he wasn't cheap; he was generous. I wasn't finished milking this cow. I was just getting started.

Brooks typically sent me one- or two-word texts. This one read, "ty." My heart skipped a beat, and not in a good way. What was he thanking me for? Is he being facetious by thanking me for peeing on him, or is he thanking me for such an incredible night in between the presumably dry sheets? Despite feeling uncertain and divided, I went with the simple and safe response: "You're welcome."

How could a man in such a vulnerable position possess such an incredible amount of control over me? I granted him permission to govern my every action. He laid down the law. He ruled the roost, even though I was not in his roost. He owned me, yet I didn't own any piece of him.

He defined whether our communication was open or closed. Our escapades were all conveniently wedged into his schedule. I never denied or forwent a request on his part to meet up. I was on beck and call. My dignity had perished along with my self-respect. I continued to allow other people to dictate my life and my happiness. I wanted to please Brooks. I couldn't say no. Just like that little girl who wanted to please her father. The cycle continued.

CHAPTER 8

Wet Dream Chaser

The first sexual encounter that I remembered occurred one week later. Brooks remained astonishingly apprehensive. He kept making plans, then backing out. I concluded that he was not a serial cheater. His cold feet and constant jitters were not the idiosyncrasies of a seasoned con artist. Honestly, I didn't care. He was still a shady con artist in my eyes. He was a pig and a fraud. He defrauded his wife into believing that he was loyal. He scammed his own children into trusting that he was a devoted father. He portrayed the quintessential father figure, but he was a sham. I was the only person on this earth who knew this man's secret, except for the hotel staff. I felt so incredibly important, yet so small. I manipulated this man's life in such a sinuous fashion, yet I was nobody. We built absolutely nothing together, except a compilation of memories that were only existent in the minds of two people. I felt cheap. I was bogus, just like Brooks.

I checked into the Pod 51 hotel in Midtown. I had already downed three shots before I left my apartment because I needed liquid courage for this type of assignment. I didn't know what to expect. Well, I did know what to expect: a creepy old man with peculiar requests. The reality was, I needed alcohol every single time I got intimate with anybody. I wasn't fully comfortable with my body. I was awkward and uptight while sober, yet adventurous and fearless while drunk. Just the thought of this man's weathered, creased body, wrinkly butt cheeks, and hairy body parts made me fearful. I was about to embark on an enterprise that would repeat itself almost daily for the subsequent year.

When I opened the door to the abnormally microscopic hotel room I was suddenly jolted with bewilderment. Why was Brooks so cheap? He could afford the St. Regis, yet we were in a room that could barely accommodate two people.

Brook shortly barged into the room, frantic as usual. He had that "outside" smell to him. I was a smidge turned off until I pictured wads of hundreds. That excited me. Perhaps just as much as vodka.

He urgently slammed down the blinds as if a private investigator was spying on us with binoculars from the adjacent corporate offices across the way. He proceeded to demand that I jump in the shower to lather, and to ensure that my perfume was no longer aromatic. He was also overthrown when he noticed that I was wearing makeup. He made it crystal clear that makeup was forbidden. I had neglected this request for my own vanity. After all requirements were reluctantly met, we stripped down to our birthday suits.

He leaned over to the nightstand and grabbed a plastic CVS bag full of goodies. He sprinkled the contents onto the bed where we were stationed. There were Sour Patch Kids, Burberry Brit perfume, condoms, and most importantly a dozen airplane bottles of liquor. The assortment included raspberry and lemon-flavored Sky vodka, vanilla-flavored Smirnoff, and six miniature Johnnie Walker Blacks. He cracked one open and knocked it back. He threw the empty bottle on the floor and grabbed another one. He cracked it open and devoured that one too, faster than the previous. I was already tipsy, but that didn't stop me from guzzling two of the bottles myself.

Brooks was no spring chicken. His body featured pockets of fat along his waistline, which complemented his scrawny toothpick legs. He lacked any muscular definition in every part of his body. Tiny black hairs shaded almost sixty percent of his body. He later informed me that shaving would be suspicious. In other words, his wife would wonder why he randomly started shaving at forty-three years of age. We didn't want her to speculate so it was imperative that he remained all-natural. He was an all-natural chicken. This was unfortunately at my expense. Those little hairs got everywhere. They were in my clothes and on my skin. They even inhabited my mouth. Fortunately, they were dark so you could see them.

Brooks ripped open the bag of Sour Patch Kids and shoved a handful into his mouth. He then pulled me in for a kiss. He opened his mouth and baby birded the entire contents into my mouth. I didn't think it could get any weirder. Was this some sick, perverted fetish? Or was Brooks just super wasted? Fortunately, I was intoxicated enough to dubiously go with the fucked-up flow. Plus, Sour Patch Kids were my favorite candy. I swallowed the bits and pieces. They tasted better than what would traditionally be swallowed during a sexual encounter. This was a perk.

Brooks was inexplicably eccentric in his lovemaking. His motions were jarring and spasmodic. He resembled a limp doll that was partially mechanical. He took intermittent pauses in which I made sure he was still breathing and not passed out from drinking too much.

Ten minutes later, the deed was concluded. I immediately became aroused as I fantasized about the wad of hundreds that he would leave on the nightstand. I thought to myself,

Easiest $1,000 ever.

His fantasy was my nightmare, and in the blink of an eye it was over. As Brooks shuffled out the door in a panic, I jumped into the shower to erase my sins. My body felt contaminated and my soul felt tarnished. I had just touched a man who belonged to another woman. He made a lifelong vow to this woman and in less than an hour sabotaged and annihilated the basic principles of marriage.

I was unsure of my role in this wreckage. I was the willing participant in this shady scam. I wasn't cheating on a loved one or hurting any children, but I was cheating myself, my integrity, and my morale. I was cheating society as well. I was *that* girl that other women couldn't trust with their husbands. I had no respect for others and consequently had no respect for myself. I don't even think I had enough consecutive hours of sobriety to feel any remorse, repentance, or empathy. My thoughts were broadly self-centered. *What do I have to do to get what I want?* Drinking numbed out any residual feelings of compassion and regret.

Drinking every single night is problematic for that reason. Even if it is just a couple of beers, alcohol still affects the way your brain processes emotion by masking your feelings. I not only utilized alcohol to deal with emotions, but I also used it to manipulate existing ones to feel more happy, confident, and social. Processing feelings in a raw, controlled, and sober mental state is challenging. It involves a sense of stability that I was lacking in my early twenties. Alcohol was the easy way out. Alcohol was the *only* way out.

Alcohol was how I learned to make love. I was a virgin until I was twenty years old. It was also at that age that I had my first drink. That age proved monumental for me. The first time I had sex I was under the influence. Alcohol lowered my inhibitions, obviously. It also hampered my anxiety, fear, and insecurities. In my mind, I was a better partner while intoxicated. These feelings affected how my sex life unfolded. In my head, drunk sex was the *only* sex. The high from the alcohol made me believe that sex was more euphoric than it actually was. Those were my expectations. I felt like I needed to drink to have "good" sex; the two went hand in hand. They were a packaged deal. It wasn't until later in life that I learned how to separate the two. After this delineation, sex became love-making.

CHAPTER 9

Beauty and the Beast

Brooks went from texting me every two days to every two hours. I became increasingly confident in our relationship. We were three months into our whirlwind affair, and I felt like I was piloting a plane with no training on how to land. I was ascending smoothly, yet rapidly. It was only a matter of time until I encountered turbulence. Even if I did maintain control throughout the bumps, I was still unfit to land. I could only predict a crash landing; I just didn't know when I would run out of jet fuel.

My emotions were imploding. I had no intention of falling in love, especially with a man who was twenty years my senior. I was powerless. This wasn't supposed to happen. I was supposed to use and exploit *him*. I wasn't supposed to be the one at the end of this narrative with a broken heart.

Over time, Brooks became less of a monster and more of prince. He had little gray hairs that speckled his naturally dark hair. He wore bags under his eyes that indicated his diligence and devotion to his hedge fund. He even downsized his gut when he started using the stationary bike at the gym. He updated his old-timer spectacles and even developed a slight sense of style in his everyday clothes. Suddenly, Brooks wasn't so repulsive. He was kind of cute. He was my quirky, mysterious finance nerd. Except for the fact that he wasn't mine. He was very much someone else's.

I wanted to spend more time with him. I got agitated and angry when he would ditch me for his family, as I grew increasingly possessive. He owned me and I rented him by the hour. I was an expensive whore. We sipped scotch, smoked stogies, and played on the adult playground. Our time together was intense and exhilarating. I fantasized about this man all throughout the day. I imagined running into him on the streets of New York. I imagined kissing him in elevators, and I envisioned our life together in the future. I was in full-fledged delirium.

On January 22, 2013, I wrote this entry in my journal:

I love this city. It oozes wealth and success. The soaring skyrises remind me that there are no limits; money is boundless, and my bank account feels bottomless. But it is not. Brooks is not permanent, he is transient. He comes and goes. This angers me. I feel like an accessory, an accent to Brooks' life. My world revolves around this man, he is my lifeline.

For every wealthy Wall Street guru is a struggling young artist trying to pay rent. I don't know where I fall in this spectrum. I'm fastened in between this world of affluence and destitution. I have money, yet, I have nobody. Money is not the cure for this loneliness. It's a reminder of my solitude.

I'm just a cocktail waitress with a college degree. I make more money than the average, tenacious junior executive but I don't work hard for it. When you don't work hard for money, it feels worthless. It's just paper. My money felt like blood money.

I live freely, and I live hard. I'm stable and unstable at the same time. I have never felt this before. Perhaps, my life appears stable from the outside, but my mind is highly unstable. It's invigorating. I thrive off this vulnerability. I'm sick.

I'm in this twisted relationship with a married mad man. From what I know, he's 43 years old, has two boys, one wife, owns a hedge fund and lives in the Beekman Towers. Oh, and he has a dog named Gretta. He is dark-haired, witty and very unwise. I like him, and he likes me. Our weeks consist of meeting at hotels, at his discretion. I have no strings, no family and essentially no attachment to anyone in this city. My only obligations and prerogatives are this man.

Brooks cannot say the same. He has a life; he is burdened by a family and he has strings tightly attached. He has places to go and people to see. I'm okay with this. I love a man with constraints and prior engagements. It feels right, it's what I deserve.

I fear commitment. I'm able to attach myself to this relationship while simultaneously enjoying my own independence and *freedom. My time belongs to me, and only me. Nothing is expected of me. No dinners, no phone calls, no guilt sex. This is my ideal, fucked-up relationship.*

I think I'm in love with this man.

I got out of work at four this morning. I rushed home and stuffed my suitcase full of lacy bras and panties. He is obsessed with the color white.

I ran into Duane Reade, picked up a box of condoms and mint Trident and arrived at our usual hotel on 39th Street.

I had two hours to spare. I cranked up the heat and jumped into the hot, scolding shower. It was so alleviating in this ten-degree weather. I sat on the tile floor of the shower, just contemplating and awaiting Brooks' arrival.

The thoughts in my head are running faster than the gushing water from the spout. Why is this such a thrill? I'm an accessory to infidelity, should I feel guilty? Instead, I feel a sense of innocence and power. I feel sexy. I know Brooks is going home to his wife every night. I don't know if it bothers me or not. I know he fantasizes about my body all day. Perhaps, his wife possesses his heart, while I possess his mind.

I love seeing him walk through the door dressed in a white, long sleeved, buttoned-up shirt. This morning, he was sporting a scruffy black sports coat. He looked inviting and marginally worn out. Of course, he was tired. He spends every waking hour tending to work and family.

Does his colossal success yield a get out of jail free card? Did he get a hall pass every few years? Was Brooks entitled to his fantasy? Or is this a midlife crisis? I don't care, this was my crisis as well. I'm building a life in this city and I'm predicting a catastrophe, a deadly crash.

We both need each other. I relied on his advice, monetary support and companionship. He relied on my free spirit, beauty and sex. We love being together. He deserves to feel good. I'm not one hundred percent sure what I deserve, but in this moment, I feel spoiled.

Brooks is selfless in bed. He is specific with his needs. He loves touching my soft, youthful skin. I dig my nails into his back, careful not to leave any evidence of adultery. His heavy breathing, sweaty hands and body language reassures me that he's pleased. I lay there, in euphoria. I am relaxed, carefree and motionless except for my hands that are grasping his now wet skin. The taboo, mystery and scandal of the whole relationship is exciting. It sparks a fire in my soul, my adrenaline rushes. I don't know if it is the sex that is addictive or the money. Each encounter ignites a new desire. I can virtually see the stress escaping from Brooks' body. For one short hour, he becomes detached and liberated from life's qualms. He then buttons up his creased shirt and prepares to revisit reality.

Brooks just left my room and I'm exhausted. I need to get some sleep. I need to be well rested for another potential encounter later this evening. I will wait patiently because that's what I do.

Goodnight, xoxo, B

Brooks promised he would come over later that night. My heart jumped out of my chest. I was elated. I performed my usual routine. I slept until noon and went for jog around Central Park. I absolutely loved the park. It was magical and picturesque. I spent hours on the immaculate and manicured grass, just daydreaming.

I started my jog on 68th Street and Second Avenue and diverted due west until I hit the park. I needed fresh air to penetrate my lungs. They felt heavy and polluted from the cigar smoke. My body was suffering. My liver was in overdrive and my lungs were exhausted. My body needed salvation. Perhaps, this jog would serve as my redemption and my heart would pump blood to repair my organs. My body was resilient. I definitely took advantage of my youth in more ways than one.

The people in the park were all prototypes of the Real Housewives. They wore permanent smiles on their faces and flaunted their lavish labels. They portrayed perfection.

The couple jogging directly in front of me sported matching tacky gear. The fact that they were conversing, mid-workout, made me believe that they weren't really exercising at all. Did they really have to spend every waking minute together? They annoyed me.

Perhaps I was exhibiting jealously of their irrefutable bond. They had something meaningful and concrete. I pretended like I didn't want that type of relationship. I convinced myself that archetypal monogamy was overrated and always unsuccessful. Expectations would consistently be unmet, and disappointments would be frequent. I clearly avoided this type of commitment to protect myself from discouragement and failure.

My relationship felt safe in the moment. But was it really? Just because I wasn't committing to monogamy didn't mean I couldn't get hurt. In that moment, insecurity and grief engulfed my mind. I struggled to defend my relationships against my own intuition. When I got home, I was agitated. I wanted to eradicate the thoughts that I perpetuated during my run. I needed to defend my relationship against my intuition, and I needed to reassure myself that I was happy.

It was five o'clock somewhere, so I poured myself some raspberry-flavored vodka into a rocks glass. I took three sips and then smacked my lips together. The taste was potent yet comforting. A warm, fuzzy feeling engulfed my senses. I immediately felt cheerful and lively. Vodka was the antidote for melancholy. It never failed to cheer me up. It made me happy, and I wanted to feel happy all the time. I never wanted to feel any lows. I couldn't handle low.

I sat in my apartment and binge-watched *Sex and the City*. I fantasized about my future with Brooks. I pictured him sitting next to me, caressing my legs. His presence was soothing and sexual. His absence left me feeling abandoned, alone, and angry.

Alcohol filled that void. Vodka was my cornerstone and my rock. It was the pillar that I stood on. It never abandoned me. It filled me with the warmth and comfort that I desired. It propped me up when I felt down and never misled me. Alcohol was my security. It always satisfied my expectations.

It was Friday night and I was sitting on the couch twiddling my thumbs for three hours. Brooks was historically flaky on Fridays, especially. He was Jewish and it was Shabbat. He was seldom able to break out on a Friday night, but I still clung to hope. It was becoming increasingly evident that I would be spending the night alone, again. I imagined Brooks sipping wine with his wife, watching movies with the kids, and munching on popcorn. I was jealous.

I pictured his wife as this troll. This made me feel better. I envisioned this tall, lanky brunette with broad shoulders. She had small breasts and a butt flatter than a pancake. She wore reading glasses, which aged her like ten years. She had no sense of style; she wore muumuus with tennis shoes and never wore a drop of makeup. She was the anthesis of me. She came from money and she was humble and courteous. Perhaps, she was *too* kind.

From day one, Brooks firmly refused to disclose his last name, where he lived, and any personal details that would humanize him. He literally stated that he was protecting his family and his identity. In that moment, I acknowledged his request while hysterically laughing in my mind. What a thoughtful, loving husband. He was just a classy man protecting his family from the woes of reality. He was just as delirious as I was. He was engaging with a twenty-three-year-old girl, literally inviting her into his life. He was flagrant and foolish. The year was 2013. I obviously Googled his phone number and was able to obtain his address, his occupation, his kids' names, his wife's name, and even his political views. This all materialized within a matter of minutes. I didn't even have to stalk the man.

Once I realized I was flying solo on that typical Friday night, I started gorging on booze. I literally devoured as much alcohol as I could in the constraints of the evening. This was a classic Brittany move when I had nowhere to go and no people to see. This was my cue. I could drink until I blacked out and pass out on my couch. My adrenaline started to pump, and I pounded another shot.

My anger toward Brooks quickly dissipated, along with all other feelings. My sadness and solitude were no longer present. I wasn't jealous of Brooks' wife anymore. In fact, she was a distant memory.

I started taking selfies and posting them on Facebook. I scored at least fifty likes and that made me feel worthy. I felt beautiful and loved again. I needed the admiration of strangers to get through that night. I was crumbling and vodka was the glue, holding me together.

I was starved. I had literally starved myself all week so that I could binge on food all weekend. That was my mode of operation and it was a weekly occurrence. My therapist called it an eating disorder, but I preferred the term "fasting." I didn't like labels.

I pulled up the dinner menu on my new computer that Brooks subsidized. I spent an hour scanning the menu because I wanted to make selections that I wouldn't regret. I saved up my appetite all week and this was my time to indulge. If I did eat during the week, I usually purged. Digesting food on weekdays was very uncharacteristic of me. It represented a lapse in judgment and willpower on my part. I couldn't afford to gain a couple pounds. My life already felt frustrating enough. Extra weight would crush me. I needed to maintain control of my life and restricting my food intake was the only way I knew how.

I ended up ordering a breakfast combo with bacon, chicken fingers with French fries, fried mozzarella sticks, and an extra side of honey mustard and ranch. I threw in a slice of cherry cheesecake to ease my sorrows. The total was $34.57 for one person and I was thoroughly impressed. Money was no object anyway. It grew on trees. I knew there was more where that came from. I was greedy and insatiable.

I never saved one dime. In my mind, my money was dirty. It was tainted. I acquired it and spent it even faster. I would deplete my bank account immediately after every deposit. I was addicted to shopping and spending money. When I was younger, I consistently reminded myself that money could buy happiness. Then why was I still miserable?

My food arrived right before I was about to black out. I could feel my legs weakening and my balance tottering. My sense of smell was dwindling, and my eyes were losing focus, my telltale signs of intoxication. I had to restart the episode of *48 Hours* twice already because I kept losing the storyline. I couldn't concentrate. I kept forgetting basic details that were crucial to the mystery. I threw in the towel.

I flipped to the Food Network because it required less thinking. This was my favorite channel to watch when I was drunk. It was stimulating, yet mindless. It complemented my high.

I ripped open the Seamless bag and devoured my breakfast food first because I didn't want my over-easy eggs to get cold. The bacon was a little too underdone, but that didn't stop me from inhaling it. Next, I munched on a mozzarella stick, dipped in ranch. The chicken tenders were exceptionally crispy and delicious. The fries were well-done, my favorite. I emptied my saltshaker onto the contents of the food and consumed everything. I dipped tenders in ranch and sticks in honey mustard. I was the queen of dipping and sauces were my wealth.

The cheesecake tasted a few days old, but it was still edible. It wasn't rancid or anything. Even if it was, I was so drunk I probably wouldn't have noticed. I sat back on the couch and noticed a ketchup stain on my rug. There was also cherry topping all over my throw blanket. I was a catastrophe.

In all this calamity, I had forgotten why I was sad in the first place. Indulging in food and alcohol was my resolution. Binging completely took my mind away from my anguish and solitude. It kept my body and my mind occupied and engaged. I got so wrapped up in the instant gratification that my emotions were put aside. They were silenced and hushed. Just the way that I liked it.

Food initiates the reward system by releasing dopamine, which signals pleasure in the brain. Once this high was depleted, I was back to square one. I could feel the copious amounts of food expanding my stomach and it was torturing me. I was in agony. I had over-capacitated my belly with breakfast, lunch, dinner, and booze, all in one sitting. I felt disgusted with myself. I glanced at the ketchup stain on my rug and became nauseous. I hated myself. In that moment, I felt like I was six hundred pounds. I felt like a slob and I felt worthless. I wanted to be empty again.

Bulimia destroys the body. It wreaks havoc on the digestive system. The bile that is forcefully emitted from the stomach is like poison. The acid tears up the throat, leaving it raw and exposed. I can attest to this. My throat was regularly raspy and sore. I also suffered from acid reflux. The sphincter, which controls the esophagus, becomes weaker, forcing acid back up into the esophagus. I was never regular; I went to the bathroom every three days. I trained my body to eliminate food the same way that it was consumed—through the mouth. My colon and intestine functions were abnormally delayed while my stomach was in overdrive. My body was a dysfunctional piece of machinery.

The acidic properties of stomach bile also deteriorate tooth enamel, which causes tooth decay. Bulimics typically demand and require more dental work than your average joe. Despite these staggering consequences, I chose to roll the dice. Since I became bulimic, I've only had two cavities. This low number reassured me that I was immune to the statistics. It encouraged me to continue damaging my body. I felt invincible. My smile was intact, and my body was usually on-point.

I darted to the bathroom and utilized the sacred toilet to purge my sins. The artificial red color of the cordial cherries, floating in the bowl, forced me to flush prematurely. I continued the craft of puking until I could feel nothing else in my stomach. I was empty, and I felt cleansed.

My memory got fuzzy shortly after I purged. The last thing I remembered was sipping vodka straight out of the bottle because the glass that I was using had the remnants of food floating in it. I said "Fuck it" and grabbed the whole bottle.

I drank alcohol six out of seven nights of the week. I seldom remember brushing my teeth before bed. I never really got ready for bed, like a normal person. I was consistently too incoherent to adhere to primitive hygienic regimens. Most nights, I was too inebriated to recall even getting into bed. Half the time, I never made it. I spent countless nights passed out on strange beds, foreign couches, and ambulance stretchers. Waking up in the hospital was all too familiar.

The following morning, I woke up in my roommate's bed; thank God she was out of town for the weekend. I hastily scoured her space for any evidence that would suggest that I had been in her room. I couldn't remember a damn thing from the night before and I wondered why I chose her bed over my own. This was just another episode in my running of drunk antics.

An hour later, I collected myself enough to run down to CVS for some fabric cleaner. I was making a valiant effort to erase the stains that speckled my roommate's outdated couch. Last night's condiments were painted all over it; it was my canvas. The final product was a hideous piece of furniture splattered with ranch and honey mustard. It was appalling.

As I opened the front door, I noticed a bag of food dangling from my doorknob from the outside. When I opened up the contents, I found a spaghetti dinner accompanied by an unbuttered roll. I didn't remember ordering this additional midnight snack. I signed into my Seamless account and confirmed that the meal mysteriously hanging from my doorknob was in fact mine. I must have been shitfaced because I would never have ordered marinara sauce. I preferred white sauce.

I threw the Styrofoam container into the microwave for two minutes and proceeded to engulf the pasta dish. I was happy as a clam. Food was always there for me. It turned my frown upside down. Brooks had disappointed me the night before, but food had pulled through and filled the void. It always filled the void.

I used to hate when people would tell me that I didn't understand what it was like to be addicted to food. I *was* addicted to food. The only difference between me and a six hundred-pound lady was the fact that I threw up my calories while the heavy person digested it. I don't know what's worse. I'm pretty sure that carrying around five hundred pounds of extra baggage was exponentially worse. The six hundred-pound lady probably has better teeth, but

I had a flatter stomach. Regardless, we were two peas in a pod; the overweight lady was just a bigger pea.

Food gave me a high, a rush of adrenaline. I fantasized about the explosion of flavors in my mouth. Once sugar or salt grazed my tongue, I was off to the races. My body craved more; I couldn't stop. I lived for food; it was the love of my life. Alcohol was also my soulmate. We were a love triangle.

CHAPTER 10

The Super Alcoholic

Brooks was mysterious and elusive. He would pop in and out of my apartment during unusual hours. He was a raccoon. He scurried around during the wee hours of the night, feeding on trash and wreaking havoc. I was the trash—the garbage that he sniffed out. His bizarre behavior, especially during the daytime, led me to believe that he was rabid. I was playing with a sick, rabid raccoon.

I loved my raccoon. He was cute and fluffy. His beer belly was my favorite body part. It protruded from his delicate frame and jiggled when he paced. He never walked; he scooted. He always looked like he was in a frazzled hurry. He had places to go, people to meet, and money to make.

Brooks hated when I conversed with other men. He sat at the end of the bar like a hawk, watching my every interaction with other patrons. One night, he barged into the bar later than usual. It was around 11:30 p.m. when he nearly tackled a feeble, old man with a cane for the very last open seat at the end of my bar. He threw a medium-sized FedEx package onto the bar to claim his territory. The package looked important, but I didn't ask any details. He was a private man and he probably would have lied anyway. Brooks started signaling my attention like an idiot. I clearly noticed him after he instigated a ruckus with the old man carrying the cane. I could tell that he was drunk because he never hand-motioned me. He was usually low-key and there was nothing subtle about the gesture that he had just made.

My heart was smiling. I loved seeing his generous face. I knew that I would be walking home with at least a thousand dollars. It was like winning a large sum of money on a scratch-off ticket. In fact, it was better because I didn't have to claim anything. My prize was instant. I assumed that his wife was out of town based on the tardiness of his visit and his intoxication level. He was a nine out of ten, and I'm not talking about his looks. He was a five out of ten on *that* scale.

I greeted Brooks with my usual napkin on the bar and "What can I get you?" He responded, "Black on the rocks and a Double Chateau." I already knew what he wanted but I deemed it necessary to appear as if I didn't know the man. We were strangers to the outside world. We didn't know each other, and we certainly didn't have sex the night before. My coworkers would beg to differ, but I shared my winnings with them so they kept their mouths shut.

I could tell that Brooks was getting agitated. He poked and prodded me. He joked, "Why don't you just go home with your boyfriend over there?" He was referring to Elias, a Greek man who was a regular at the bar. We partook in flirtatious banter and small talk. Flirting was my bread and butter; it was how I earned my money as a bartender. It was essential, just like alcohol. Brooks didn't understand. He reminded me how much money he was funneling me and asked me why I would even waste time mingling with anyone else but him. He was acting possessive; he was wasted. I couldn't just snub the other patrons. They were paying customers and they anxiously anticipated my attention.

At first, I thought Brooks was joking about the flirting. Twenty minutes later, I realized that he was being very serious. Smoke came out of his ears and offensive words came out of his mouth. He was out of control. Every innocent bystander noticed the fiasco. I needed Brooks to peacefully exit the bar before he caused more of a scene. This man was unbelievable. He climbed into his king-sized bed every night with his wife and he was angry at me for flirting? What universe was I in? This was absurd. This was a grown-ass man, acting like a greedy little bitch. He needed to go. I wanted my money and I wanted him gone.

After giving him a piece of my blown mind, he stormed out of the bar without paying his tab. I was furious yet reassured. I noticed that he left his stupid package. It was wedged between the corner of the wall and the sticky bar top. I assumed that he would pull a 180 and storm back in so I didn't touch the package.

I needed more alcohol. I was approaching sobriety—a state of mind that I dreaded. I generously treated myself to an adult beverage. I poured a Grey Goose and soda, with more vodka than soda. I chugged the entire glass. It was gone in sixty seconds. The brain freeze didn't faze me. Chills crawled up my spine and the hairs on the back of my neck perked up. My head got light and my knees got weak. My stomach burned and my heart turned warm and fuzzy. My body felt as high as my spirits. My married boyfriend became an afterthought. The only thing on my mind was alcohol. I consumed about four more drinks throughout the course of the night. By 4 a.m. I was flying.

While closing the bar, I vaguely remembered the bulky white package that Brooks had left on the bar four hours prior. It was clearly not on the bar anymore. I tried to recall its whereabouts, but I was unsuccessful. I thought, "Hopefully it wasn't a package of money," and then I chuckled. I took that back. I *did* hope he had lost a package of money. He was being an asshole and he deserved it.

I counted the money in the register, wiped down the bar top, and blew out the candles. A normal person would have gone straight home. But I was an alcoholic, so I wandered over to the after-hours bar next door with Brenda, my coworker. We walked through the door and noticed the usual suspects sitting at the bar. They were all industry people who had just gotten out of work. The five of us took a shot of Fireball. The last thing I remember was holding Brenda's hand and giving her a peck on the cheek. We got affectionate when we were drunk. We were best friends, and this was our way of bonding. If we were lesbians, we definitely would have married each other. Unfortunately, I was strictly heterosexual, and I think she was too.

I woke up in the morning with more than a headache. It was a generalized body ache. I was hurting. I was on top of my covers, still wearing the tiny, black, halter-top dress from last night. It reeked of musty cigar smoke and regurgitated scotch. I aggressively rubbed my eyes and then noticed my hands and fingers covered in black mascara. I was livid that I didn't wash my makeup off before passing out a few hours earlier. I changed out of my dress for pajamas and walked into the kitchen to assess the damage.

I noticed that the kitchen window was wide open, a visible dirty shoeprint on the tile, and chunks of dirt that resembled soil. The shoeprint was too large to be mine. I pondered for a moment. I didn't remember a damn thing from the night before. Regardless, I was positive that I didn't bring a man home. I became frazzled. Based on the evidence, I reconstructed the scene and deduced that a crime had taken place. The open window, the shoeprint, and the suspicious soil were clues left behind from the perpetrator. I put my investigator hat on and concluded that someone had broken in. I scoured the tiny two-bedroom apartment for any missing valuables but came up short. Despite my lack of concrete proof, I dialed the police.

A whole hour later, I hear a solid knock and NYPD was at my door. I felt tense and hungover. The man was a pudgy midget in a uniform. He looked more like a mailman than a police officer. He apologized for the delay.

Apparently, he was downstairs conversing with my nosy superintendent, Chuck, for fifteen minutes. Chuck was an alcoholic who was sober for over twenty years. He was a diehard AA member who hit a meeting at least twice a day. I'm pretty sure he was one of the founding fathers, back in 1935. He quoted the Big Blue Book and recited the twelve traditions on a daily basis. He was certainly a "trusted servant" of the self-governing entity. He identified as an alcoholic and he made sure that every tenant in the building knew it, including me.

Chuck was already pulling security footage from the window where the perp had supposedly gained entry. I should have been relieved that we were going to apprehend the culprit, but I wasn't. Once Chuck got involved, I became uneasy. My roommate and I were already on his bad side. He constantly complained of marijuana wafting from our unit. We vehemently denied the allegations based on the man's sober status. I didn't think he would buy the medical marijuana spiel. It was a drug and he believed that if you do drugs, you die.

I was shaking in my boots. I couldn't remember the events that took place the night before and I wasn't sure what Chuck was going to witness. When I heard him clamoring up the single flight of stairs, my heart dropped out of my chest. His cheap rubber boots were pounding each step and his pace resembled a stomp. I could tell that he was enraged. He busted through the door without a knock and couldn't wait to tell me that a man had crawled through the window around six in the morning. I took a sigh of relief.

He then proceeded to elaborate. He said, "It looked like your coworker. From what I can see from the grainy footage, you were fumbling, looking for your keys for a good twenty minutes outside of the front door. Then, your 'friend' climbed up and into your window." Apparently, I had lost my keys and my coworker who had kindly walked me home had crawled through the window to unlock the door.

I was speechless. My face turned as white as a ghost. I was mortified. I cocked my head and squinted my eyes in confusion. I responded, "Oh, ha. So that's what I did last night?" The cop was the only one that snickered. Chuck was a stoic statue. I had no other option but to plead guilty. There was nothing to confess since I didn't remember anything, but I did acknowledge that I was blacked out.

He gave me the look that my dad used to give me when he was disappointed. Chuck was judging me. He started ranting about Alcoholics Anonymous. He reassured me that I wasn't too young to admit that I had a drug problem. Between the marijuana and the drinking, he was on to me. He was more intuitive than Judge Judy. He was equally as intelligent but slightly more forgiving. I was the defendant, being sued for neglect. He pounded his gavel and passed judgment. I listened to his shtick for nine minutes before apologizing profusely. He understood that I was an alcoholic, but he failed to convince me. I pretended like I was reevaluating my behavior and nodded my head up and down. He had a valid point, but I was too hungover to heed any of his advice.

I resorted back to my safe space and took a shot of Limon Ketel One that my roommate's dad had left in the cabinet. He had tragically passed away, so I safely assumed that his alcohol was fair game. My throat burned and I immediately felt better about the whole scenario. I rationalized my unfortunate situation by chalking it up to normal drunk shenanigans. I questioned, "Does shit like this happen to everyone who drinks?"

Brooks called me four times in a row as I was passed out on the couch. On his fifth attempt I answered with a mumble. My eventful morning had caused me to forget about my eventful night. Brooks sounded frantic. His voice cracked and his tone was stern. He didn't even greet me with a "hi." He spit out, "Do you have my package?" I responded confidently, "Nope." He asked me if I was joking and I facetiously said, "Yeah, I threw it away after you acted like an asshole last night." When he raised his voice, I realized sarcasm wasn't the strategy to utilize in that moment. I admitted that I didn't have it and that someone must have snagged it after he left. He proceeded to inform me of the package's importance. I shrieked, "Why in the hell were you lugging around a package of cash?" He abruptly hung up. I didn't care. I was mad at myself for not pocketing the package for myself. After all, he had walked out on his tab.

I sat on my couch for the rest of the day, analyzing Chuck's powerful words. I was outraged that he had inserted himself into my personal life by suggesting I had a drug problem. The reality was: I had inserted myself into *his* life. I had wasted two hours of this man's time and energy. My egotism and discourtesy were indirect consequences of my alcoholism. Instead of feeling remorse, I felt irate. I was a girl with zero repentance. I walked over people and wasted their time. The only sacrifices I made were for the bottle. I chose alcohol over everything else. I protected and defended my drinking at all costs. I was codependent.

CHAPTER 11

The Phone Call Girl

My bank account was thriving, and my wardrobe was booming with designer labels. I was giving away my shifts at work and I was spending copious amounts of time with my lover. Working became fruitless; I was making exponentially more money with each interaction with Brooks. Thursday was thousand-dollar Thursday and every other day he was giving me upwards of $600. My pints of flavored Smirnoff shifted to handles of Ketel One. My freezer was perpetually stocked with Johnnie Walker Black and Grey Goose. I was a functioning alcoholic. My life seemed perfect to the outside world. I had my family, my friends, and even my coworkers fooled. Or at least I thought I did.

It was the morning of February 14 in 2013. My phone started ringing at 8:45 in the morning. My head was spinning, per usual, and I exhibited signs of intoxication from the night before. I ignored the first call because I thought it was my mom. I was not in a sound and coherent condition to convince my mom that I was sober. I dozed back off into a trance.

My phone rang again. I was now under the assumption that this was an emergency. Someone needed me. I unwillingly and regretfully answered my phone. The woman on the other line spoke swiftly and softly. Her accent sounded British, but I could have been entirely off base. The charming woman asked me if I knew a man named Brooks Epistein. My ears immediately perked up like a dog with a whistle. I sobered up quicker than a fat kid chasing an ice cream truck. I sat up straight, I cleared my throat, and I responded, "Is he okay?" My initial speculation was that he was dead. The woman's voice resembled that of a caring nurse. Perhaps, my phone number was the last to correspond with Brooks'. I honestly believed that I would become the recipient of sobering, yet somber news. Perhaps he was in a car accident or had a heart attack and was in the hospital.

The woman replied, "He's okay. How do you know him?" My tongue twisted in a knot and eventually tied. I was speechless. I spilled a few words, but they were nonsensical, "Uh, I don't know, um, why?" The lady then confidently made the statement, "Brooks is my husband."

My heart sank and my stomach dropped. All of my organs dropped down to the cold, hard floor. My eyes opened wider than a double-wide trailer. I bit my bottom lip as hard as I could, and I scrunched my nose tighter than a facelift. My mouth dried up when I attempted to piece together my rebuttal.

She spoke first. I had zero words to say, and she had a million. She asked me how I knew him. I said, "We are friends." I could tell that she smelled bullshit.

I explained to her that I was a waitress at Merchant's and we were "literally just friends." Just a couple of pals, who liked to shoot the shit. She wasn't buying it.

I anxiously adhered to the blatant lie. I kept repeating "We are just friends" like a broken record. Those were the only words that I could scrape together. Regardless of my unshakable stance, the woman tried long and hard to bend my ear.

I knew I was lying, and she knew I was lying. My nose was growing longer by the second and sweat was literally dripping down my face. Her next question was odd. She asked me if I had ever touched him. My response was epic. "Ew, no, he's old and gross." I didn't understand this lady. She kept prodding me. Did she really think I was going to spill the beans that easily?

I felt like I was on a hamster wheel and this woman was never going to let me off. She sensed my frustration. Her final words were, "Stay away from my husband."

Those words singed on my brain like hot coal for the following three years. Who was *she* to tell *me* to avoid her husband? I was pretentious and haughty. For so many years, I did what I wanted to do, regardless of the consequences. I was an entitled, little brat.

I immediately texted Brooks four little words: "Your wife called me." He called me back about twenty minutes later. He was more distraught than I was. He was a Tasmanian devil; he was frantic as fuck. He couldn't even take breaths in between each word. I was way too sober for that shit.

He put me on a Ferris wheel. He went around and around. His exact words were, "Deny, deny, deny." We were just friends, end of discussion. He told me that if she discovered any secrets from our affair that he could never talk to me ever again. And, that's how the conversation ceased.

I was devastated and pumped at the same time. I honestly didn't believe that I would never see him again. He couldn't live without me. He needed me.

My adrenaline was in full fucking throttle. Every possible outcome of this scenario crossed my mind. There were two ways that this crisis could play out. The first scenario was in my favor. The wife would kick Brooks to the curb; I would swoop in and offer my shoulder to cry on. The two would get a divorce and she would obviously take half of everything that he owned. I would move into the Beekman Tower and the two of us would live happily ever after.

The second scenario made me cringe with fear. The wife would threaten Brooks with divorce. In desperation to save his marriage, he would disown me. I would be dead to him. This scared the shit right out of me. In my heart, I didn't think he was physically capable of staying away from me. He was a man with many needs. I knew one thing for certain: Brooks was addicted to sex; he was not mentally or physically capable of quitting cold turkey. He was a junkie.

Brooks made it clear that I couldn't call or text him under any circumstance. I begrudgingly conceded and waited for him to call me, which he eventually did.

The following day, Brooks called me at noon, on the dot. He was slurring his words; he sounded inebriated. I got aroused. He advised me to meet him at the Salvation Taco Bar. I had just rolled out of bed. I tossed my hair up in a messy bun and threw the same clothes on that I had worn the night before. It took me less than ten minutes to get to the agreed location. It took another ten minutes for me to down two shots.

Brooks stumbled into the establishment. I barely recognized him. The bags under his eyes were even more conspicuous and his facial hair was untamed. He looked like he hadn't slept in a week. He looked like he was on a crack bender. I didn't look much cleaner. I was hungover, as usual, and my face was puffy from binging and purging the night before.

Brooks told me that his wife had taken a flight out to Denver to reevaluate their marriage. He made it apparent that the only reason he was meeting with me was because he was wasted. He repeatedly combed his fingers through his long, unkempt hair, like a mad scientist. He resembled a person who was experiencing psychosis. He kept twitching and rocking back and forth, like a psycho.

He recycled these words: "She's going to leave me, she's going to take everything." He looked like a man who was desperate to save his family. On the contrary, he was sitting right next to me. His words led me to believe that he wanted to save his marriage; his actions led me to believe that he wanted me. I had never been this dazed and confused in my life. This reckless man was dispatching mixed messages. He was a typical man; he wanted to have his cake and eat it too.

The alcohol was flowing and so were the tears. Brooks was practically sobbing hysterically. He looked so pathetic, sitting on that scrawny barstool pouring his heart out to his mistress. I awkwardly rubbed his back and made a conscious effort to console the grown man. I remember making ridiculous assurances. I said things like, "Don't worry, we will get through this together." When he said that his wife would take half of his money, I responded, "Don't worry, we don't need money to make us happy." I can't help but laugh uncontrollably at my thought process in that moment. I responded blindly in pure insanity. This grown-ass man was clearly wasted off his ass and I was clearly delusional.

Brooks had a decision to make between love or money. He could choose me, which would cost him his fortune. Or, he could choose to stay in a loveless marriage and retain his finances.

The harsh reality: What we had was not love. It was simply sex. With that epiphany, I knew I would never see this man again.

That afternoon, we drank ourselves into oblivion. We hooked up in the Salvation Taco restroom. That would be the last time that I ever rendezvoused with Brooks. Perhaps I was saved that day. Rescued from a man more toxic than alcohol. He was poison.

CHAPTER 12

Dish of Dirt

My life was in shambles. Within a week, my bank account was back to three digits. The vodka bottles in my freezer were dwindling and my tears were running dry. I went from having it all to having nothing at all. I felt deceived and dumbfounded. I didn't know if it was the alcohol or the heartbreak, but I was certainly disorientated. I had never experienced heartbreak, and in that moment I didn't even know what I was feeling. This man was not my husband or even my boyfriend. He was fundamentally an alien to me. I was dead to him, but he wasn't dead to me. I thought about this man every waking second of every day. I compulsively checked my phone for texts and calls and I furiously looked for him while I was at work.

I fantasized about Brooks walking down the stairs into the cigar bar. I wanted so badly to see his shadow standing in the doorway. Work wasn't the same. It didn't feel right.

I drank excessively throughout my shifts. There were several occasions when I blacked out toward the tail end of the night. I was even caught stealing alcohol from the bar. I would ring in drinks that were not actually for my customers. They were for my consumption; they were for my stability and sanity. The bartender had caught on to my maneuver. I was ringing in a lot of vodka Diet Cokes, no ice. And, the only time she was concocting that peculiar drink combo was when I was working. I got a slap on the wrist and a tongue lashing. I gave zero fucks. Carrying a pint of vodka in my purse was easier anyway, plus all that flat Diet Coke was bloating my stomach.

Brooks called me from a payphone approximately five times in the subsequent three months. This pissed me off. It gave me a flicker of optimism that he still wanted me. Every time he anonymously called, he was bombed out of his mind. He was drunker than a skunk when he insisted that I meet him at this bar in Midtown. I was on a date with a repulsive, old guy. He took me to a diner on our first date. In addition, he ordered chicken pot pie. What freak orders pot pie on a first date? I pretended like I had to use the ladies' room, and I sprinted out the door, into the wind. I left that cheap creep high and dry.

I met Brooks at a venue called The Monkey Bar. This was my first confrontation with the man who had torn me to shreds. I walked into the bar area and I heard a chirping, like someone was trying to get my attention. I was more eager than embarrassed. He proceeded to signal me into the elevator. We both walked in with a group of random strangers. We pretended like we were strangers. I was acclimated to that game; we used to play it all the time. We were never seen interacting with each other in public. We were discreet, anonymous, and unsuspecting.

Once we had the elevator exclusively to ourselves, I predicted a hot make-out session. Instead, he slobbered on me, like a dog. I think he was trying to kiss me, but he was entirely too intoxicated. He muttered some mumbo jumbo and then cut to the chase. He reached into his wallet and handed me six folded hundred-dollar bills. A rush of memories flooded my dazed mind. A movie reel of our tumultuous affair flashed in my head; it was intense and fiery. I remembered all the laughs, the passion, and the heat. When I looked at Brooks in that elevator, I saw a man I didn't recognize. That fire was extinguished.

The elevator doors swung open, followed by a ding, and Brooks darted out into the haunting night. This scene looked familiar. It's exactly what I had done to my date, hours earlier. I walked home forty blocks that night feeling bitter, tormented, and misled. The only perk was my fat wallet. Why did this man keep torturing me? He kept barging into my life, at *his* discretion. This made it exceptionally more challenging to erase this man permanently from my life. He was a gnat that I couldn't shoo away.

Brooks wasn't the only gnat. His wife bombarded my phone with peculiar and personal questions, shortly after she had returned from her trip to Denver. She was unusually inquisitive. She asked me if the sex was good and if I was sleeping with other men. For a month, she prodded me for every disturbing detail of the affair. Our interactions with each other were mutually motivated. She pressed my buttons and I pressed hers harder. She demanded the facts. She was building a case against her guilty husband. I was *her* witness and *his* accessory to adultery. I was playing both sides. I provided her with all the evidence that she needed. My goal was to convince her that her husband was the devil. We both knew he was a pig, but most men were. He was more than a pig. He was the devil in disguise. He was a pervert and a predator. He was an awful husband and a monster.

Despite all these shortcomings, I still wanted to be with him. My goal was to get his wife to file for divorce. I wanted her to leave his ass. I knew this was a long shot, but it was my last resort. Why do women remain married to husbands who consistently cheat on them? Is this what unconditional love looks like? These questions haunted me.

I could understand a one-time mistake that involved alcohol. Because I, of all people, understood the power of alcohol over the human mind. Alcohol changes who you are as a person. It manipulates your thoughts and behaviors. It suppresses your inhibitions and your liability. It mutes that little voice in your head that reminds you that something is a bad idea. Everyone makes mistakes, but not all suffer the consequences.

I believe that everyone deserves a second chance. Well, most people. Alcohol is not an excuse for poor choices, but it certainly answers the age-old question regarding intentions. Alcohol distorts and alters true intentions.

Regardless, Brooks habitually cheated on his wife, like clockwork. Even with the threat of divorce looming over him, he couldn't stop. He was addicted to me.

Divorce is a scary word. Brooks and his wife had spent twenty-plus years building a family; she must have feared that loss. But is divorce really a loss? Women who support shitty husbands are the ones losing, trapped in marriages that are unfulfilling. A good woman deserves a man who treats her with dignity and respect. How could Brooks' wife accept his behavior and allow him to continue to drink? It was pure blasphemy.

Brooks and I deserved each other. We were both disingenuous, selfish, and disrespectful. His wife was none of those things. It wasn't until I got sober before I felt any remorse. I was an accessory to infidelity. I perpetuated and participated in an appalling affair. I managed to wedge myself in between a marriage and then managed to bow out, unscathed. This shitty human whom I loved was no longer in my life. The wife was the one left picking up the pieces to a shattered life.

The story should have ended there. I should have picked up my own life and walked away with a fresh start. Unfortunately, I did not make it out unharmed. I no longer had Brooks in my life, so alcohol became the star of my show. It outshined everything and everybody. My alcoholism monopolized my life.

I could no longer afford my rent. I was living with a roommate on the Lower East Side. When we had signed the lease four months prior, I was rolling in the dough.

Paying $2,100 for my bedroom was a piece of cake. Plus, Brooks had assured me that my rent was always covered. I was now in a pickle. I made about $2,000 a month as a bartender, which meant that if every dime went to rent, I was still short $100. I was fucked. My roommate, Mike, was also strapped for cash. We were both fucked. We developed a plan that would require renting out my bedroom via Airbnb. This accommodation left Mike and I sharing his bedroom and the small living room. This modification was miserable. I could not tolerate the situation, unless I was drunk. We were exclusively drinking buddies, and that's how I wanted to keep it. When Brooks jumped ship, Mike swooped in, romantically. Our new arrangement was *his* ideal accommodation, unbeknownst to me.

Mike was a fifty-year-old man who had previously worked as my manager at Merchant's Cigar Bar. Our friendship flourished throughout the years. He even dated my sister. He was sarcastic, charming, and generous with the few dollars that he had. He was also mysterious. He was a successful business owner throughout his thirties but lost his restaurant because of shady dealings. He owed over $100,000 in taxes and even filed for bankruptcy. Acquiring the managerial position at Merchant's was his fresh start. It was the quintessential position for any man in pursuit of beautiful girls. It gave him the opportunity to work alongside gorgeous cocktail waitresses wearing six-inch heels and short dresses. This was any man's dream job.

Mike was shady. He was divorced with two or three kids. He hadn't seen his children in years and failed to pay child support. He was a classic deadbeat. I was now sharing a room with this deadbeat. We drank every single night to erase the fact that we were both losers.

The first thing we did when we arrived home from work was pour a drink. I was compelled to drink around Mike. I hated him less when I was wasted. On this night, we both entered the apartment around nine. Mike's friend was staying in the Airbnb for the time being. He was a six-foot-tall ogre who took one shower a week. He was always cooking his special soup on the stove that reeked of rotten seafood. It consisted of frozen calamari rings and cans of tomato sauce. Coincidentally, he was a broke alcoholic as well. He would buy handles of McCormick vodka and pre-mix cocktails into a Vitamin Water bottle. Our freezer was literally filled to the brim with bottles of pink Vitamin Water, all mixed with shitty vodka and calamari rings.

I got home and immediately cracked open a bottle of the spiked Vitamin Water. I cleared a space on the floor and sat down amidst an array of disheveled clothes and garbage. I played *Grand Theft Auto* until I could feel my vision get blurry from the booze. I abandoned the controller and settled on television with my two roommates. We watched YouTube and music videos for two consecutive hours. The last thing I remember is chugging from my Vitamin Water and watching *Epic Rap Battles* on YouTube.

I woke up in Mike's bed, nothing out of the ordinary. We frequently shared a bed, due to the unusual circumstance. We were just friends, or at least that's what I thought. I noticed I was wearing a different shirt than the one I had on the previous night. I thought that was bizarre. I was also not wearing underwear, so I harmlessly surmised that I never put them on to begin with. This was not an uncommon occurrence.

Fortunately, I was still drunk from the night before, so I speculated that I had fallen asleep around four in the morning. I peered into the mirror. My hair hadn't been dyed in months and my split ends were conspicuous. My face looked like a blowfish. Aside from the bloat, I had gained fifteen pounds, which I attributed to my unsuccessful eating disorder. I was getting so intoxicated at night that I passed out prematurely, before I could purge my food.

The hot pink tank top that I was wearing was smothered with stains and embedded with crumbs. I felt utterly disgusting. I felt fat, hideous, and grotesque. My hygiene was poor and my effort was nonexistent. I shuffled to the bathroom, kicking shoes and bottles that littered the wood floor. When I turned the door handle, it was locked. I cursed out loud and released a sigh, loud enough that the neighbors could hear. When the ogre opened the door, I got a whiff of air that was rotten and potent. The ogre pooped at least three times a day, making the bathroom a danger zone essentially the entire day. I needed a gas mask and a hazmat suit. I sat on the stained couch, waiting patiently for the smell to subside. I was too nauseous for that shit.

The ogre sat next to me and tried to make small talk. He commented, "You had a fun night last night." I was perplexed. I assumed he was being facetious. I had blacked out and I was curious. I asked, "Did we do anything fun last night?" He let out a chuckle and a snort. He responded, "Well, you and Mike did."

My heart sank, per usual. I sternly asked, "What do you mean?" He said that Mike and I hooked up. I replied, "Are you fucking serious?!" He leaned back on the couch in hesitation. He said, "What do you mean? You don't remember?" He proceeded to tell me that Mike and I frequently shared more than the bed. He got defensive. He also disclosed that I repeatedly professed my love for Mike, but only when I was drunk. Allegedly, I would say things like "I love you" and "Let's get married." I choked up and ran to the rancid bathroom to throw up.

When I stepped out, Mike was standing there. I started to tear him up. I yelled, "What the fuck! You know I don't have feelings for you. You dated my sister!" All the pieces of the puzzle were falling into place. Mike knew damn well when I was in a blackout. He also knew I would never get with him while sober. I deduced that he would wait until I was in a blackout and then place moves on me. He took advantage and I felt extremely violated and it wasn't often that I felt violated. I usually took accountability for events that transpired when I was shitfaced and this was not my fault. He was the last man in my life whom I actually trusted.

This man knew that he was off-limits to me. He exploited and offended me, for his own sexual gratification. He was supposed to be my friend and I was in shock. I couldn't trust anyone. Most of my friends in the city were solely drinking buddies and I considered Mike to be more than that. He was my brother, we always fought, and I hated him. I had thought his greatest shortcomings were his bad breath and terrible grammar; I had no inkling that he was a predator. Three days later, I stuffed most of my clothes into three twenty-gallon trash bags and moved the fuck out. I swiped every spiked Vitamin Water out of the freezer and tossed them into my bag.

As much as I loved alcohol, I hated it. It hijacked my mind, leaving my body vulnerable to strange men. I hated men even more. They were all dishonest, perverted, and sacrilegious. Men were out for themselves; they were more selfish than women. All they thought about was sex. It was disgusting, and *they* were disgusting. They all had ulterior motives; they were all cheaters. A man's mind was more twisted than mine. It's a mind that cannot be trusted.

CHAPTER 13

The Wife Comes to Life

Two months after my escape from the hell on 12th Street, I began to exhibit signs of healing. I had moved in with a friend on the Upper East Side and was paying less than a thousand dollars for rent. I completed my first stint in a hospital detox unit, which forced me to slow down on my drinking. I was exercising regularly and gradually shedding my vodka weight. I still thought about Brooks every day, but I was still functional. It was a Thursday evening and I had just returned from a run along the West Side bike path. I was in my new apartment, searing tilapia on the stove. My phone rang. It was a random number but I reluctantly answered it.

I heard Brooks on the other line, drunk as a skunk. My heart skipped a beat. My ears started ringing and my legs nearly collapsed. He swiftly rambled two inaudible sentences. I caught the words "Bar and Books" and "seven o'clock." It was like Morse code, but I fully comprehended his message. I honestly didn't think twice about my decision to meet him there. I was utterly broke, and even though I didn't need Brooks, my bank account did. I was desperate for cash and this was a deliberate sign from God.

I chose an outfit to impress. I wore a strappy red and tan striped tank top, with no bra. It loosely dipped all the way down to my belly button. I used double-sided tape to prevent a nip-slip. When I turned the right way, you could see my glistening belly button ring. My black skirt barely covered my butt cheeks. It was too short to wear wedges, so I chose strappy sandals. I was ten pounds down, and I felt confident yet confused. This man kept popping into my world with no regard for my well-being. I knew he hadn't changed.

I arrived at Bar and Books, which was a cigar bar that happened to be a couple doors down from Brooks' residence. I grabbed a vodka and soda and a Johnnie Walker Black and sat at a table, farthest away from the bar. It was discreetly tucked into the back corner of the venue. The lighting was dim, and the music was Frank Sinatra. It was intimate.

Brooks barged into the bar and nearly hurdled the steps. I stood up to give him access to the interior of the booth. He was googly-eyed as he scanned my open cleavage. He wasted no time and placed his hand on my thigh. It felt surreal. I had thought I would never feel the touch of his hand on my bare skin ever again. He kissed my lips as he shifted his hand higher. I almost felt violated. He kept telling me how much trouble he would be in if his wife found out. He started berating me for divulging every secret to his wife. I tensed up and shrugged my shoulders. He had no idea what hell he had put me through, and I had no clue what hell his wife had put him through. We were even.

He stood up to access his back pocket. He slammed $400 down on the delicate table and stumbled up the stairs and out the door. Before I had a chance to even sip my drink, he was a phantom in the night. He was elusive.

I sat there for a couple minutes, processing the string of events. I peered out the window and a goldendoodle caught the corner of my eye. I had seen that dog before. A year prior, Brooks had shown me pictures of his family dog with his head out the window of his white Jeep Rubicon. I pieced two and two together and realized this was the same dog.

Two minutes later a woman stormed into the bar. I knew exactly who this woman was. She sat down about three inches from me. In a British accent she asked, "Was Brooks here?" It was a rhetorical question. She knew that he had been here. His half-empty scotch was still planted on the table and I'm sure she could smell the traces of his Bleu de Chanel cologne.

I perched up against the back of the booth. I was still sober, and very terrified. She was a furious middle-aged woman. She was like a lion protecting her cub and I felt like a child who was about to get scolded. She was classy in her buttoned-up, collared shirt and shoes that resembled Sperry's. She was taller than me and carried a little more weight. She wasn't full-figured. She epitomized class and status. Her hair was peppered with grays, and her wrinkles decorated her all-natural face. She had big brown eyes and her eyebrows slanted down, which gave her this look of melancholy. I pitied her.

All her counterparts were dining with their husbands and she was face-to-face with her husband's mistress. I was impressed with her tenacity. She demanded that I hand over my phone so that she could browse my texts. I retracted and responded, "Hell no." I wanted her to think that Brooks was still actively texting me. We bickered back and forth like an old married couple until we were interrupted by an intruder who had just walked in. He said that there was a dog tied up outside on the lamppost that had gotten loose.

The wife's final words were, "Stay away from my husband," as she stomped away and out the door. I felt my adrenaline pumping faster than a speeding bullet. I wrapped my sweaty fingers around Brooks' glass and tossed his scotch down my hatch. I proceeded to polish off my vodka and soda. I was in cardiac shock. My heart was racing faster than a racehorse's. I second-guessed my own actions. I regretted my noxious attitude. I had behaved like a juvenile, catty, and cheeky little girl. I felt like white trash. I felt like a whore. She was put together, decked in a buttoned-up blouse. I was a hot mess, exposing my chest for everyone to see.

Half of me wanted to cry and the other half felt empowered. I possessed this power over Brooks and I still felt relatively present in his life. The attention that I'd received that evening was enough to make any addict satisfied. I was angry at Brooks yet flattered that I still crossed his mind. Once again, the wife had his heart while I had his mind. He was definitely still consumed with me or at least thought about me.

One week later, Brooks called me again. This time from a stranger's cell phone. I safely assumed that he was intoxicated. He propositioned that we meet up at Bar and Books. Was this a set-up or a sting? Upon arrival, I vividly imagined the wife sitting there at the same exact table, waiting to tear my head off.

Mercifully, when I opened the door, I noticed Brooks in the corner of my peripheral vision. He was sitting at the bar with two empty scotch glasses stationed in front of him. I scrolled over and plopped down on the neighboring bar stool. The grown-ass man was toasted. This was unequivocally the most inebriated I had ever seen him. He announced to the entire bar that his wife was overseas, during the holiday.

Then he proceeded to hurl wads of cash at me, like I was a stripper. After a couple words were exchanged, he stood up unsteadily. He walked five steps, like a baby giraffe first learning how to walk. Shortly thereafter, he tumbled onto the red, velvet couch that graced the back wall. There was no way this man was making it home alive.

I quickly assumed the role of a good Samaritan. I grabbed his arm and insisted that I walk him home. I felt like I was helping my hundred-year-old grandpa walk down the street. The only thing missing was a walker. He popped into the bodega next door for a coffee and we continued on our way. His lukewarm coffee was splashing out of the sip hole as it spilled down his white shirt and black denim jeans. We approached the Beekman Towers, where he insisted I come upstairs. I wasn't in the mood to explain to his children why their father was so drunk. And, I wasn't in the mood to clarify who I was.

This decision was progressive for me. It took all the restraint to refuse his offer. I wanted so badly to ride that elevator up to the thirtieth floor and generate mayhem. Perhaps that would be the straw that broke the camel's back. Unfortunately, I was too sober for that shit. I reluctantly stood there, on the corner of 48th, and watched Brooks stagger into the extravagant entrance to his luxury residence. That was the last time that I would ever see Brooks again—stumbling off into the night.

CHAPTER 14

Intoxicated and Loveless

A year passed by and I steadily got my shit together. Not totally together, but I had moved on from Brooks. He had left a distinct scar on my heart and fortified my preconceived notions regarding all men—they were pigs. Because of these lifelong scars, I made a commitment to myself to seek men who were the complete opposite of Brooks. I dated guys who were respectful, decent, and most importantly loyal.

It was the summer of 2015 when I made the decision to move back in with Avi, in Queens. We had left off on a rough note back in 2013 but I reassured him that I had matured. More importantly, I could hardly afford the thousand dollars that I was paying to live on the Upper East Side. I was soliciting myself on sugar daddy websites simply to pay my bills. In other words, I was meeting up with older, wealthy men in exchange for financial support.

This exchange was degrading and humiliating. I was relying on creepy old men to pay my bills. I was desperate. I was subconsciously seeking another Brooks, which I never found. All the men were cheap and revolting. I couldn't do it anymore. I was at my wit's end. I ceased all interactions before I strangled one those men with my bare hands. I didn't want to go to jail so I moved back to my fellow Asian community.

Life went full circle, and there I was, back in Queens. It appeared as if I had regressed, when in fact I hadn't. I was very much moving forward. I had wriggled my way out of a deep, dark hole that Brooks had thrown me into. He then shoveled dirt into the hole, but I didn't suffocate. I could hardly breathe, but I'd survived. Although I sprouted, I wasn't fully mature. I wasn't even close.

 Shortly after moving, I started working at Sidebar, a "Gator bar" that was notorious for the scantily clad servers, typically decked in sports jerseys and daisy dukes. I had shriveled down to a hundred pounds; my tan was on-point and my blonde locks were freshly dyed. I fit the mold of the stereotypical hot bartender and was hired on the spot.

At the time, I was immersed in two active addictions, alcohol and an eating disorder. I was binge-drinking on weekends in the Hamptons. Then, on weekdays, I was running upwards of ten miles a day and eating downwards of a hundred calories per day. I was making no effort to curb my food cravings. I was binging and purging every other day. I had mastered my eating disorder. I knew exactly what to put in my mouth in order to preserve my skeletal physique. I was overexerting my body, so I felt obligated to fuel it. I powered up with raw spinach, pickles, and celery sticks and splurged with the occasional tomato.

One day, I caved in and ate one whole, triangular, multigrain tortilla chip. It made me anxious. I imagined my thighs chafing and my abdomen accumulating pockets of fat. I entered my usual "fuck it" mindset and began gorging myself with food. I ate leftover Persian food, chicken kebobs, and doughnuts. I obviously polished off the remaining tortilla chips. Meat and dense carbs were historically more arduous to throw up, but I accepted the challenge. Everything was fair game for a seasoned bulimic like me. I dashed up the squeaky stairs and purged every bit of food until I was left lightheaded and featherbrained. I brushed my teeth and splashed cold water on my face to deter swelling. I felt high. Most importantly, I felt in control.

Obsession is the hallmark of addiction. Whether it's food, drugs, or sex, your brain becomes fixated on feelings of pleasure that the substance or behavior elicits. It's a process that normal people will never comprehend. The anticipation and the build-up become stimulating and irresistible; it's a part of the high. Just thinking about food or alcohol would rouse those tiny butterflies in my stomach. Blood would barrel to my head as I became instantaneously dominated by an overwhelming sense of excitement and emotion. Yes, emotion. My absence of genuine feelings in other aspects of my life was a consequence of my preoccupation with my drugs of choice. Food and alcohol superficially satisfied my emotional needs by evoking comfort, joy, and instant gratification. My desires were insatiable, and I practiced indulgence on a daily basis.

I couldn't just eat one chip. I couldn't just have one drink and I couldn't just run one mile. Everything I participated in was performed in excess. I couldn't stop. My brain perceived pleasure with no interference. It never registered satisfaction. It never signaled fulfillment. It was quite the opposite; it compelled me to keep going. It convinced me *not* to stop. My craving for over-indulgence wasn't necessarily a choice. I didn't choose for my brain to send me these conflicting signals. Why couldn't my mind just tell me when to stop?

Two months into my career at Sidebar I started drinking on the job. It was a Thursday night when my coworker and I shared a bum bottle of Tito's Vodka. We drank from the chic glass bottle every hour. The restaurant was lifeless, and boredom creeped into my ailing mind. My girl and I were cracking jokes and philandering with the few patrons that we had. I was buzzed and feeling gregarious when Sidebar's marketing manager, Drew, stole a seat at the bar. I pumped the brakes on my alcohol consumption, while Drew stepped on the acceleration. He was full throttle. He was pounding Bud Lights like they were going out of style. We exchanged flirtatious banter and partook in intimate conversation. We were hitting it off.

Drew was a good one. He was respectful, dependable, and bashful around pretty girls. He was boyfriend material. He was sarcastic, witty, and intelligent. The only pitfall was his stout physique and average looks. He possessed these bug eyes that were aggressive and eerie. He wasn't an ogre, but he certainly wasn't Brad Pitt. The moral of the story: I wasn't attracted to him. Luckily for him, I was drunk. My beer goggles were fastened tightly around my eyes. Four drinks in and he became easier on the eyes. He invited me to the bar across the street called Shades of Green. This bar was a hole-in-the-wall. The alcohol was cheap, and the patrons were even cheaper. I would eventually rename the bar "Shades of Black" because of all the times I had blacked out there.

Drew and I sat at the bar and immediately downed shots of Fireball. Unbeknownst to him, I was already completely in the bag. The last thing I recalled was the dusty blue floor in the shabby ladies' room. I didn't even remember walking out of the establishment.

Apparently, I did make it out of the restroom because I woke up in someone's bed. When I opened my swollen eyes, I rolled over like a sausage and noticed that I was alone. I contemplated whether I had gone home with Drew, and my heart stopped beating. Perhaps I had gone home with someone else; I hoped it wasn't a female. I glanced around the room at the crooked, unframed pictures and I knew this bedroom belonged to a male.

Whose bedroom was this? It was a mystery that I had been forced to crack many times before. As I curled up with the blanket, I observed a two-foot bong lying next to the nightstand. Instantaneously, I knew that this was Drew's because he was a marijuana connoisseur who participated in daily smoke-out sessions. I didn't know Drew well, but I did know he was a pothead.

I was impressed with his apartment. It was two-bedroom gem in a luxury building, complete with a doorman and a gym. It was ideally situated near Second Avenue in the heart of Murray Hill. It was also located about fifteen blocks from Sidebar. I fantasized about how convenient it would be to live there. I could literally stumble home from work after a cumbersome night of partying. I wanted to live there.

I started dating Drew because I wanted to be treated right for a change. His apartment was the icing on the cake. He was an authentic gentleman. He listened to things that I said and gave me sound advice regarding life decisions. He was so caring and lovable. He was certainly not a ladies' man; he was more of the class clown. He was the eternally single guy who could arouse laughter in any crowd.

Our coworkers smelled something between the two of us and I basked in the attention that we received. Because I was slightly out of Drew's league, his buddies were more than excited for him. This was his first relationship in over three years, and he'd scored a diamond. I was cubic zirconia, shiny and dazzling for a few months until my partner discovered I had a drinking problem. From the outside, I had my shit together. I was an avid runner and a hard worker. I could also hang with the boys and could hold my own. My sarcasm was on-point and so was my body. At this point in the game, Drew and his friends had no idea I was an alcoholic. I didn't even know. It was my deep, dark, and coveted secret that I protected for many years. I defended alcohol to ensure that it was always incorporated into my daily life.

Within three weeks, I was partially moved into Drew's quaint little apartment. My game plan was unfolding on cue. My intentions weren't entirely pure, but I would ultimately pay the price. Every night with Drew was the same. He was certainly a creature of habit. We would run down to the neighboring bodega, grab a chicken cutlet sandwich and a twenty-four pack of Bud Light, and retreat to our fortress. The remaining night consisted of drinking beer and watching baseball or *King of Queens*.

I loved Drew as a friend. We jibed because we had the same intelligence and sense of humor. Our biggest discrepancy was the fact that he was awfully generous and I was awfully selfish. That man showered me with love, compassion, honesty, and loyalty. I was his priority while alcohol was my priority.

I maintained functionality as an alcoholic for at least two months before I lost my job. It was a Wednesday in November when I woke up with a screaming hangover. I was depressed and dissatisfied with my routine. I was sick and tired of the monotonous life that I was building with Drew. I lacked passion and an overall desire to be with him. I couldn't stand to watch one more baseball game. I didn't even like baseball.

I realized I was rapidly catching a case of the "fuck-its." The symptoms were classic and irrefutable—a lack of desire to work, socialize, and function normally as a human being. I looked in the mirror and noticed my thighs were kissing. Makeup was smudged all over my face and I looked like a crack whore. I was too hungover to embark on a journey to the liquor store. It was too daunting. I needed alcohol to erase these disturbing and depressing thoughts. So, I did what any seasoned alcoholic would do: I ordered a bottle through an online delivery service. The minimum delivery purchase was $50. I had two choices. I could either buy one nice, healthy bottle of Grey Goose or I could get two or three plastic bottles of the cheap shit. Once again, I did what any professional alcoholic would have done. I chose option B. I had to work later that night, but I chose to disregard my obligations. My job was placed on the back burner.

The disease of alcoholism convinced me that I could have a couple drinks before work, sober up, and then head to work like a normal, functioning human being. This was a classic Brittany move. I always told myself I could handle a couple drinks before I had somewhere to be or something to do. One hundred percent of the time I ended up drinking too much and ghosting the responsibility. My brain would convince itself that *this* time would be the exception. I was always the exception in every scenario. In reality, alcoholics were never the exception.

I would cut myself off at two drinks and I would be responsible. My intentions were pure, but my alcoholism dictated my intentions. Once I started drinking, I couldn't stop on my own. My brain would tell me that nothing else was important. And no, no one was holding a gun to my head forcing me to drink. My brain was persuading me to drink despite negative consequences. I didn't choose that persuasion; I didn't choose that diseased brain. I wanted a brain that would tell me stop. I wanted a brain that would listen to my intuition.

When the doorbell rang, I was already two Bud Lights deep. I grabbed the bag of goodies and hid one of the bottles in the top cabinet above the refrigerator. I gave myself a heavy pour and withdrew to the living room. I watched three episodes of *My 600-pound Life*. I dozed off and curled up on the couch with my bottle of vodka, like a baby with its milk bottle. When I woke up around 1 p.m. I was feeling in the dumps. The alcohol did not punch me in the face like I wanted it to. I was far from happy. It didn't bestow an incredible burst of energy and it certainly didn't give me irresistible food cravings.

My sadness turned to anger. I stomped to the kitchen and took a couple more shots. I stood there and looked at this oversized, plastic bottle of alcohol. I needed to get rid of this evidence. It was not optional; it was a requirement. How could I rationalize drinking half a bottle of vodka in the middle of the day? I couldn't hide the bottle in my secret cabinet above the refrigerator because I would lose easy accessibility and I would need the bottle later. My wet brain needed to think lucidly. I opted to pour the vodka remnants into a water bottle. Not just any water bottle; I poured it into a flavored water bottle. Drew despised flavored water because of the off-putting aftertaste. This maneuver had zero cracks. I was confident that my vodka was safe and secure in this deliberate little bottle. Drew would never touch it and therefore would never know. I felt sneaky. I loved the deceit of my alcoholism. It gave me vitality and life. It made me feel smart.

After I emptied the bottle of vodka, I tossed it down the trash chute—the black hole of garbage. My evidence was disposed, into the abyss of other tenants' innocent garbage. I returned inside and started eating the buffalo mac and cheese that was left over from the night before. I felt less depressed while eating. Unfortunately, I couldn't just eat all day. I looked at the clock on the microwave and it was already two o'clock. My heart sank. I didn't want Drew to come home from work. His face annoyed me. He thought our relationship was perfect, but it had its cracks. It was severely flawed.

A typical night looked like this: He would arrive home from work and hit the bong. Then we drank beer and ordered food. We sat on identical, side-by-side recliner chairs and held hands as we watched TV. I despised this. I was uninterested, bored shitless, and only cared about drinking more alcohol. Drew knew I loved drinking but misunderstood my fixation and dependence. He also turned a blind eye. He never once told me that I should quit. He needed a drinking buddy, and if I were sober, then he would have to give up his beloved evening ritual of Bud Lights. He constantly rendered comments about slowing down or not drinking so fast. All his wisecracks were taken with a grain of salt. He was an alcoholic too; he was the pot calling the kettle black. He wasn't going to tell *me* to slow down. He had no clue I was already half in the bag by the time he got home from work.

The last thing I remembered on that Wednesday afternoon was lying on the loft couch watching trash TV. I woke up in Drew's bed around midnight. I was befuddled. Did I go to work last night? I had no clue. Drew heard me rustling around in the sheets and woke up. He was pissed. I was his girlfriend and consequently my actions were a reflection on him. He had attempted to concoct an excuse for my absence, but Gregory, my manager, hadn't bought it. Drew broke the news to me right then and there, at midnight, as we lay in his bed.

He evidently couldn't wait to break the news that I had been fired. I think he thought that it would be a wake-up call. He thought that I would quit drinking and reassemble the pieces of my life that were in shambles. He didn't know that I was a full-fledged alcoholic. He had no inkling that I drank despite negative consequences. In fact, losing my job only fueled the fire. It was a catalyst to drink even more.

From that point on, Drew babysat me. Our relationship went from a friendship to a parent-child relationship. I couldn't understand why he continued dating me. I was a complete shitshow. I was a mess. I was never sober around him. We would spend the day together and I would devise plots to escape for fifteen minutes so that I could run to the liquor store.

One time, I told Drew I was going to the gym. His ears perked up because he thought that I was turning a corner. He thought that I was putting down the bottle and picking up the barbells. This was a rational presumption. When I did practice sobriety, I became addicted to exercise. I displaced one addiction for the other. In those bouts of sobriety, I would compulsively work out and become obsessed with being thin. For Drew, *this* addiction was the lesser of the evils.

Unfortunately, alcohol was still very much my drug of choice on that day. I strutted to the liquor store and bought four airplane bottles and a pint of vodka. I trekked to the building's gym where the real trickery materialized. I jumped on the treadmill and pounded the rubber until my face turned beat red. Then I pounded two airplane bottles. I sat on the workout bench and called my mom. I restricted my phone usage and only called people when I was buzzed. I couldn't handle a sober conversation. Twenty minutes later, I splashed water on my face and drenched my shirt to replicate sweat. I was bubbly and effervescent as I rode the elevator to the twelfth floor.

Drew rarely smelled alcohol on my breath. His sense of smell was below par. Perhaps he did get alcoholic whiffs, but he kept his mouth shut to avoid confrontation. This was common. He was fearful of me. He rarely spoke his truth. He was dedicated to ensuring my happiness. I don't know if it was because he thought I was so incredibly hot or because he genuinely loved me. Either way, it was a disservice to himself and me.

Alcoholics often manipulate people they love. We deliberately engage in relationships where we can acquire the upper hand. I was a professional. I had Drew wrapped around my finger. He was a highly functional alcoholic. He was never staunchly capable of forgoing his nightly case of Bud Lights and I knew this and took advantage. He thought he was controlling my alcohol intake. He strictly counted my beers and prohibited hard liquor in the apartment. I ignored and bypassed these stipulations. Therefore, I gained all the control. It was all a sick game that Drew negligently played. His actions were driven by love. My actions were driven by my addiction. My addiction reigned over our relationship, leaving Drew paralyzed and vulnerable.

CHAPTER 15

I'm a Freaking Alcoholic

Three months after losing my job, I got back on the wagon. I flew home to Florida where I could dry out for two weeks. I demanded space from Drew. It was my only means to achieving sobriety. My brain convinced me that I needed alcohol to be around him. I was a bitch when I was sober, and he didn't deserve that. Drying out was hell on earth. The temptation to drink was forceful and vigorous.

My mom was in the dark about my withdrawal. She owned a cleaning business and was gone most of the day. She took advantage of my presence and kept requesting my assistance with the household chores. I wanted to drink so badly but I stuck it out. I couldn't let my mom see what shape I had put myself in. I slapped a smile on my face and pretended like I was not withdrawing. I remember puking when I undertook the task of scooping the cat litter. My stomach was sensitive, and my brain was cloudy. My mom would ask me questions that I couldn't answer. My brain function was at half-capacity.

The most severe symptoms were my uncontrollable shakes and night sweats. I avoided human interaction at all costs. When I reluctantly conversed with my mom, I held my hands together, tightly grasping my fingers, to evade visible trembling. I took frequent showers to erase the salty sweat that kept drying on my parched skin. Every night, I discreetly washed the sheets to exterminate the puddle of sweat that my body excreted throughout the excruciating night. For a week, I couldn't sleep, eat, or think normally. My muscles ached and my mind throbbed. It was torture. I told myself, "This is the last time I'm ever going to experience withdrawal." I was never drinking again.

I returned to New York with a newfound admiration for sobriety. I wasn't planning on staying sober forever. I was going to drink occasionally in moderation. I was spending most of the week back in Queens to dodge the temptation of Drew's fridge, jam-packed with Bud Lights. We met for sushi on Fridays and went shopping on Wednesdays. He annoyed me. His bug eyes stared relentlessly at me. They were laser beams that were provoking me to drink. Those eyes were powerful.

I didn't have a job lined up when I flew back from Florida. Browsing Craigslist became my daily routine. I looked for restaurant jobs, preferably not bartending. It was too risky. I didn't think I could find a job in advertising because

I didn't feel competent. Serving and bartending was my only skill. It was straightforward and I was comfortable. A *real* job would have required way too much effort. I was insecure with my abilities, so I settled for the restaurant industry.

I stayed at Drew's whenever I had a job interview in the city. Otherwise, I was back with Avi. I could live without Drew, but I couldn't live without his conveniently located dwelling. Even though I was dry, my brain still functioned as an alcoholic. I continued to use and abuse people.

Alcohol damaged my righteousness. My demeanor was unassertive, and I couldn't handle emotions. I stayed with Drew a few days at a time partly to avoid confrontation. I felt bad for Drew. He loved me so much and I didn't want to break his heart. He was gracious and compassionate. He was also too emotional. I was selfish and made the calculated and cold-blooded decision to continue our relationship despite not loving him. Ironically, he was my charity case. I felt so incredibly bad that I had sucked him into my web. I wish I would have trapped a man like Brooks; he deserved pain. Drew didn't deserve to be hurt by a girl like me.

Two weeks after returning from Florida, I landed a job at Brother Jimmy's across the street from Madison Square Garden. It was a comfortable hike from Drew's, and I fell in love with my manager, Jessica. The job required extensive knowledge of the food and drink menu. I was three days into the job when a coworker recommended that I taste each cocktail, for professional purposes. My heart wanted to politely decline the offer, but my alcoholic brain seduced me. It convinced me that I could successfully sip each drink without tumbling off the wagon. I tasted the Charlotte Tea, the Kentucky Mule, and the Southern Sangria by sticking a straw into the glass while holding the other end. The minuscule amount of alcohol that I consumed tasted like heaven. I hadn't eaten and I could feel a little fire ignite inside of my stomach. The burn empowered me. I felt instantaneously ignited. I wanted more.

My natural train of thought directed me to the neighboring liquor store, like a horse being led to water. I was not forced to drink; I freely and voluntarily drank from the bottle as I walked the twenty blocks back to Drew's apartment. I was feeling positive and peppy. For the first time in over a month, I anticipated Drew's arrival. He swung the door open and I gave him a big hug. He was astonished but he didn't hate it. For the first time in two months, we hooked up.

I woke up with a nuisance of a headache. I needed to be at work at 10:30 a.m. Drew was fumbling around with his bong when I slipped past him and into the kitchen. I opened the fridge and witnessed an imaginary halo around the shelf that was chock full of Bud Lights. I needed the hair of the dog. It was my remedy. One beer would rejuvenate my otherwise sluggish and lethargic body. I swiped a beer and wrapped it in the towel that I was holding. I jubilantly skipped to the bathroom, beer in hand. I cranked the shower on and simultaneously ran the sink faucet. As I flushed the toilet, I coughed and cracked open the Bud

Light. I waited for Drew to say something and heard radio silence. I was in the clear. I drank my beer and lathered up my loofa.

On my way to work, I made a pit stop at the liquor store. I snagged a pint of Smirnoff, only for security. I would only open it if I got too shaky. I didn't think I would, considering I hadn't been drinking for consecutive days.

When I arrived at work, I performed my usual duties. I made the homemade tea, refilled the sauces, and set the table placements. The drab and wet weather was deterring restaurant-goers. It was nearly noon and I had served only one table. My buzz had waned, and I was vexed that I had made only $15.

A case of the "fuck-its" were casually creeping in. I felt consoled when I made the ruling to crack my stash wide open. What was I waiting for? I felt foolish for not consuming my potion earlier. Who was I kidding? I chuckled. I grabbed my purse that was underneath the server station and shuffled into the unisex restroom. I didn't have a spare bottle of Vitamin Water to mix with the alcohol. Instead, I emptied out a water bottle into the sink and poured the entire pint in. I held the pint high to ensure the slender part of the stream would enter the tiny opening to the bottle. I was a qualified and skillful pourer of alcoholic beverages. I didn't waste one drop of the liquid gold. I was a proud pourer.

Throughout my dry spells, I constantly hushed my brain because of the relentless fantasizing about drinking. I would stonewall my feelings, which inevitably left me in a cold turkey situation—staying sober solely because of willpower. My brain was programmed to crave alcohol, yet my intuition reinforced me that I couldn't drink. I knew the difference between right and wrong. I chose not to drink simply to avoid roadblocks. Sobriety was vital throughout major life changes; i.e., getting a job, visiting family, moving, and attending events. These experiences were crucial in my perceived functioning as a human being. The moment I hurdled or surpassed these junctures, my alcoholism screamed louder. It went from a dull murmur to a thundering roar. It ravaged me when I was vulnerable. It reminded me that I could have just one drink when life steadied out. Because of this cycle, my early twenties resembled a model of ebbs and flows—episodes of sobriety, followed by a lengthy bender. There was no in between. Drinking once or twice a week wasn't in my repertoire. I either binged every single, consecutive day or didn't drink at all. I was a *true* addict.

My coworker was looking at me sideways as I shoved my purse underneath the POS system. I sensibly and naturally vocalized that I was on my period. My coworker snickered and responded, "Hah, that's what I thought." I felt an instant sense of deliverance as I shrugged my shoulders. My ability to improvise in a jam was impeccable. This was a common talent that most alcoholics shared. We had to think on our feet to combat any agnosticism while fulfilling sketchy schemes. During active addiction, we were shady as hell.

I left work that day feeling high as a kite. I stopped on my way home for some cupcakes for Drew. I got him four perfectly frosted cupcakes, decorated in rainbow sprinkles. I also stopped at a sushi restaurant. I sat at a puny two-seater table and ordered a glass of Pino Griot. I started studying the Brother Jimmy's menu in preparation for the server test that I was being administered the following day. I was overconfident and presumptuous because I had been studying persistently for a week. When the sushi server dropped off my wine, I ordered edamame.

Halfway through the wine I made the executive decision that I was going to purge the meal. I added fried calamari, a spicy kani salad, a red dragon roll, and a Godzilla roll to my order. I rationalized and told myself that I wanted to rid all the alcohol in my stomach so that I would appear less drunk when Drew arrived home. Therefore, the food would conveniently come up with the booze. It was a win-win. That justification was a crock of shit. I didn't care what Drew thought; I was just ravenous and refused to digest all the spicy mayo that I was about to eat.

When I got back to Drew's place, I removed the little piece of tape that secured the lid to the cupcake box and opened it up to snap a quick picture. I loved Instagramming pretty food. The fluffy frosting and pastel sprinkles were like the sirens from Greek mythology. They were luring me in with their enchanting colors and moist presentation. So, I did what I normally did and I placed Drew on the back burner and selfishly ate all four of the luscious cakes. Shortly after, all of the delectable food that I had just eaten was partially digested, floating in the toilet bowl. This required two flushes because the seaweed tended to float. It was gone forever. I proceeded to wipe every crevice of the porcelain toilet with Clorox. My secret was safe.

When Drew returned home, I was passed out on the couch. Fortunately, he thought I was innocently napping. I woke up, dazed and confused. He made a comment about my red eyes and dilated pupils. In a drunken stupor, I reluctantly revealed that I had enjoyed a glass of white wine with my sushi earlier that evening. He didn't look pissed, but he certainly wasn't happy about it. I took a deep breath and sigh of relief. He got a whiff of alcohol when I did so. Thank god I had confessed minutes earlier; at least I didn't look like a liar. I proceeded to elucidate my epiphany that I had during my stint of sobriety. I convinced Drew, and almost myself, that I could in fact drink alcohol—in small doses and not consecutively.

The look on Drew's face was perplexing at best. I interpreted my reality and once again defended my alcoholism. I clarified that I was only twenty-four years old, and that it was unrealistic for me to simply quit drinking altogether. Instead, I needed to focus on moderation. Therefore, we could both enjoy our evening nightcap, just not in excess. It was as simple as it sounded. Practice self-control and put a kibosh on binging. I was a freaking politician because I sold Drew my classic alcoholic speech and he bought it faster than a melting snowcone. That night we enjoyed a case of Bud Light and no sex.

The following morning, I woke up drenched in sweat. I was just elated that it wasn't urine. My brain function felt dull and inadequate. It was normally intact and razor sharp. Actually, that was a lie; I was always hungover. I thought since I hadn't blacked out the night before that I would have miraculously woken up with no hangover. I was wrong.

I needed mental clarity for my official Brother Jimmy's menu test that was being administered in a few hours. I made the rash decision that I was going to chug a Bud Light. When I opened the fridge, I found an empty blue box that once housed twenty-four cans of beer. *Fuck* was my sole thought.

I hurriedly got ready for work. I didn't have to work an actual shift; I was solely going in to execute the test. Therefore, I had to appear only halfway decent. Drew offered to share a cab with me, but I politely yet urgently declined. I don't think he would have welcomed a pitstop at the liquor store, especially after the bullshit I had sold him the night before.

I snagged a pint of Smirnoff at the liquor store, took a swig in the Starbucks bathroom, and arrived at work with my memory intact. I felt as sharp as cheddar cheese and as buzzed as a bee. I completely aced my test. My manager allowed me to have a congratulatory drink at the bar and then I left the establishment before I got too intoxicated. I stopped at the adjacent Taco Bell. I was mingling with strangers and engaging in frivolous conversations. I proceeded to inhale a Crunch Wrap Supreme, a Chicken

Chalupa, a Nacho Bell Grande, and cinnamon churros. I was drunk off Smirnoff and high on life. I had just aced my test and I felt astute. I hadn't felt this accomplished in months. I was proud of myself. For once, I didn't hate myself.

One week later, I was still endorsing my alcoholic stance regarding moderation. Unfortunately, my actions didn't align with my words. I was bringing a bottle to work every day, solely to ride out the day. On the first day of my bender, I was drinking to feel high. Now, I was drinking to avoid the blatant trembling and the crippling cold sweats. If I were to walk into work stone-cold sober, I wouldn't be able to hold a tray, remember a drink order, or even climb a flight of stairs. I was broken. I needed alcohol to fix my impaired body.

It was a Sunday when I headed into work around 9:45 a.m., anticipating a routine pitstop at the liquor store. As I swung the corner of Fifth Avenue I noticed the "Open" sign was turned off. As I pulled the immobile door handle, I remembered what day it was. It was my least favorite day—Sunday. Liquor stores didn't open until noon. I was fucked. I arrived at work ten minutes late. I was already drenched in sweat and trembling with fear. The last bit of alcohol was being excreted through my pores as I sweated. I was losing steam, and I was losing stamina. I felt like the walls of the restaurant were closing in on me. My lungs were caving in. I was in a state of pure terror, solely because I needed alcohol. My body needed it to function. I was a robot, running out of batteries. I was dying.

The hostess sat my first table, a four-top. I walked over, feeling lightheaded and faint. When the people started rattling off their orders, I became flush and frozen. I wrapped my fingers around my pen, but my fingers wouldn't bend. They were stiff and useless. I loosely held the pen with my pointer finger and my thumb. When I touched the black ink tip to the pad, my hand conspicuously jolted. I couldn't write.

I struggled to remember the entire order, including the food. I couldn't even recall the two soft drinks that were mentioned. My brain was in a delirious fog. I felt like I was a hundred years old, with dementia. I could have sworn that I was seeing little strings attached to the ceiling. I was hallucinating. I felt unhinged and I was unraveling by the minute.

I looked out the window at the closed liquor store across the street. I felt like a prisoner in my own body. I was contained in this tiny cell, controlled and powerless. My only cure was liquor, but I didn't have the key to get it. I remember slinking into the restroom like a dog with its tail between its legs. I crouched down on the grimy, grisly, checkered floor and just sobbed. I was a fucking slave to alcohol. I would literally have killed for it, in that moment. I was a desperate, imprisoned soul—locked in a dungeon called alcoholism. I was tortured and suppressed every fucking day. I was suffering from a disease that fucked with my mind. It was the Stockholm Syndrome—I was in love with my captor. I was a hostage to alcohol, yet I exhibited positive feelings toward it. I loved, cherished, and relied on vodka. Yet, it mentally and physically tortured me and nearly killed me, hundreds of times before. Was I crazy? I needed to abandon, eliminate, and annihilate alcohol, simply to survive. It was the enemy this entire time. It was the antagonist to this entire story, not Brooks. He was just a broken man. It's crystal clear to me: I'm an alcoholic.

CHAPTER 16

Dry as a Bone

The day that I labeled myself an alcoholic was ironically the same day that I freed myself from the stigma. It was easier to admit that I was an alcoholic than to convince myself otherwise. All the signs pointed toward alcoholism. All I had to do was take my head out of the sand. When this revelation came to light, my life up to that day made perfect sense.

Every childhood memory echoed into adulthood. Every poor decision was attributed to some deficiency in character, and every uncontrollable behavior derived from my inability to adapt to changes. Maladjustment was prevalent in every aspect of my life. The problem was my lack of coping skills; alcohol was the answer. I thought it was solving problems in my life, but it was only creating them. I was trying to extinguish a fire but instead was accelerating it.

The only tool I had in my toolbox was alcohol. I grew up watching my dad model a reliance on alcohol, and I watched my mother maladapt to those inferior circumstances. During this upheaval, I was powerless. My emotions were futile, and my feelings were voided. As a child, coping meant avoiding. As an adult, coping still meant avoiding. And, I learned through my dad, the easiest way to do that was with alcohol.

Being honest with myself regarding my addiction was the first hurdle. Next, I needed to be honest with myself regarding my happiness. I knew what needed to be done. I had to cut my ties with Drew, regardless of how convenient his apartment was. This meant that I needed to be honest with him; his heart needed to be broken, sooner than later.

That day of my revelation, I didn't return to Drew's apartment. Instead, I took an Uber back to Queens where I detoxed for the next week. I explained to Drew exactly why I had gone back to Flushing that fateful day. I told him that I had been on a bender for a while and that I needed time alone to detox. "Alone" was the operative word. And, I clarified precisely what I needed from him during this time. I craved breathing space, freedom, and detachment. I didn't want him to feel too horrible, but I know he did. He couldn't grasp why I didn't just detox in his apartment. He seemed offended and a little hurt. Despite being an alcoholic himself, he couldn't comprehend my language. I needed to focus on myself. I needed to discern what made me happy, and I needed to explore what would keep me sober.

This type of exploration was stifled in the presence of a man. My thoughts became conflicting and my motives became ulterior. During my infancy stages of sobriety, men were just as toxic as alcohol itself. For so many years, I had used and abused them in retaliation for my own personal mistreatment from men. They were not people; they were pigs. This absolute and categorical mindset proved unfair to Drew. He was a victim, caught in my web of lies, misconduct, and addiction.

Ten days later, I rode the Long Island Railroad into Penn Station and met Drew at our favorite sushi restaurant, Hiroshi. I sipped hot green tea and nibbled on edamame as I undertook the feat of interpreting my alcoholism and how it affected my behavior in our relationship. In my dismay, Drew wanted to forget everything and start fresh. He was prepared to forgive and exonerate every single one of my sins, including the lying, the stealing, the cheating, and the drinking. My heart sank and my stomach nearly dropped out of my butt. Literally, all I did was blame my mistreatment and misconduct on my alcoholism and, BOOM, forgiveness prevailed. It couldn't be that easy; I didn't want it to be that easy. I wanted Drew to feel anger, fury, and rage. I wanted him to yell "Fuck you!" and storm out of the restaurant, leaving me with the bill. Most importantly, I wanted him to hurt me because I deserved it.

Finally, I wanted him to feel a sense of relief when I ended it. It was supposed to be a win-win. The drunk monkey was peeled off his back and I was liberated from any ball and chain that would affect sobriety. I needed to regain and redefine my newfound freedom. I needed my independence to explore who I was as a woman in sobriety.

Drew and I walked solemnly back to his apartment so that I could reclaim my possessions and he could reclaim his bedroom. He needed to salvage the wreckage from beneath me. I had wreaked havoc on his life for eight months too long. He deserved the peace, freedom, and respect that I had selfishly stolen from him during my reign of terror.

With Drew behind me and sobriety in front of me, I had hope for my future. I walked into Drew's coveted apartment and noticed two suitcases, a duffle bag, and a trash bag full of my belongings just staring back at me. My heart started racing and I felt a massive lump in my throat. I could feel my vocal cords swelling up and my throat felt full and tight. My body was preparing me for impending doom, and my fight-or-flight response was kicking in. I had to break out of that tiny apartment before my tear gates broke open. The clock was ticking. Drew offered to walk me downstairs. I politely declined. I was surprised when he didn't offer an Uber to Penn Station. The trash bag was loosely secured to the dented handle of the rolling suitcase, which was busting open from a broken zipper. I looked like a homeless person who was migrating from Uptown to the Lower East Side. I couldn't show any signs of distress.

When Drew missed his opportunity to call an Uber, I knew he was pissed. I was ecstatic when I concluded that he was not only bitter but mad as well. I wanted him to be furious; it made my tears hide back into their reservoir in the lacrimal glands. His anger made it possible for me to walk down 34th Street without shedding a single tear. By the time I arrived at the steps of Penn Station, my shoulder was throbbing and my heart was aching. Alcohol would have made this scenario less painful. Smirnoff was my armor. Unfortunately, I rode her until she bucked. I dusted myself off and left that horse alone. My alcoholic ride was over. The horse was dead.

Over the next two weeks, Avi and I prepared for a magnanimous move from our rinky-dink cave into a gorgeous three-bedroom duplex in Bayside. The Asians, who owned the building that he was renting from, were demolishing the space. They needed us out in less than thirty days; we were out in two. I was ecstatic. The new abode was a beautiful brick-faced gem, erected on a tree-lined street, adjacent to charming manicured lawns and pristine sidewalks. The Long Island Railroad station was less than a mile away and provided an abundance of ease. The train itself was luxurious, equipped with cozy seats, tray tables, and even power outlets for your electronics. My commute to work was a breeze and certainly a breath of fresh air. I was in heaven on earth, also called Bayside.

Drew was a far-flung memory, and my current love was this neighborhood. I didn't deserve this bounty and beauty. Perhaps this was God's contribution; he was illustrious in his support of my sobriety. God genuinely graced every stride that I took. He was present and glorious. I thanked him every day for the blessings of sobriety and bliss. He was my rock; he was my savior.

Life was surely less chaotic, living as a sober woman. My mind began to stabilize along with my life. I developed routines that were never instilled while I was drinking. I adopted a nightly skin care regime and even started bleaching my teeth. While drinking, I never remembered laying my head down on my pillow, much less washing my face. I had neglected basic healthful living.

The most radical adjustment was learning how to fall asleep. My mind was a merry-go-round of thoughts and feelings. My anxiety peaked immediately after the sun set. It was aggravated by inactivity and equanimity. I literally couldn't sit with myself and my own thoughts. Panic, chaos, and turbulence all attacked my mind like an invasive species. Apparently, the outward chaos that drinking generated was a coping mechanism. It distracted my mind from my inner demons. Alcohol was the impeccable interference between the noise in my head and my consciousness. It temporarily solved a problem, but I needed permanence. I needed to learn to sort through my thoughts, my anxiety, and my feelings. Sobriety wasn't an end game, but a gradual, lifelong practice. I honestly thought that I could stay sober with willpower. I had not yet discovered AA and was not attending therapy. I was white-knuckling my sobriety.

The new dwelling certainly kept me physically and mentally occupied and engaged. I painted my bedroom, rearranged furniture, hung pictures, and allocated decorations. I remained active even after I returned home from work. I didn't give my mind a single opportunity to wander. I was a busybody, which was a euphemism for mild OCD.

By week two, we were completely moved into our townhouse. There were no more pictures to hang or photos to frame. The house was spotless, and the yard was immaculate. I started watching TV at night, which really aided in my ability to unwind and decompress. I watched shows that were engaging and captivating. TV shows that occupied my mind were vital in fending off any anxiety and intrusive thoughts. I binged on *48 Hours Mystery*, *Dateline*, and *Snapped*. True crime shows were my creed. They tied up my brain and kept the demons at bay.

The thrill and stimulation of the big move from Flushing was in the rearview mirror. The chaos from my breakup was terminated, and the high of sobriety started to fade. The air felt dead and motionless. I needed excitement; I needed to stir things up a little. I craved adrenaline, and the plot thickened.

Spring was evolving rapidly into summer and the weather was idyllic. Brother Jimmy's was packed to the gills with tourists, and customers' tips were cumbersome and generous. The restaurant itself was undergoing a revamp, including the outdated menu. It was a Tuesday when the refurbished menu was introduced to the staff. To familiarize ourselves with the new menu items, we tasted every morsel of food. It was a revolving door of plate after plate after plate. It was fantastic and intoxicating.

We tasted fried pickles, rib tips, fried green tomatoes, southern fried chicken, Nashville hot chicken, baby back ribs, sliced brisket, and even fried Oreos. I had been eating religiously healthy for a month now and this greasy food tasted heavenly and delectable. I remembered my coworkers asking me, "Where do you put all that food? You're so small." Those words were like music to my ears. I imagined my coworkers giving me an applause and a standing ovation. I was scarfing down more food than a fat kid. I couldn't stop; I was relentless. When the revolving plates came to a halt, I felt uneasy. My stomach was over capacity while my brain compelled me to eat more.

My addiction to food was pernicious and precarious. Once the food hit my tongue, I couldn't stop eating. I binged on food like I binged on alcohol. One drink was too many and a thousand drinks were not enough. Unfortunately, this reality applied to food as well. One chip was too many and a thousand were never enough. The only difference was that I couldn't avoid food altogether. I needed to fuel my body; I needed energy. My relationship with alcohol was nonexistent, but I couldn't just break up with food. I needed to arbitrate a healthy balance. This regulation would persist every single day for the succeeding five years. Balancing food intake with an eating disorder proved intricate and sticky. Lines were drawn, lines were blurred, and lines were crossed.

When I left the restaurant, I was dead set on purging. I had no other option. I didn't want my digestive system to become overloaded and I didn't want heartburn. I stopped at CVS to acquire more food. I got multigrain goldfish, Teddy Grahams, and white chocolate-covered pretzels. I plopped down on the plushy, blue, cushioned seat of the LIRR and proceeded to rip open my goodies. As the train approached the Bayside station, I stood up and noticed that my chair was chock-full of crumbs and debris. I inspected the interior of the car to ensure my confidentiality. No eyes were on me. When I drew a deep sigh, my stomach felt tightly compressed. I didn't *want* to purge; I *needed* to. I waddled all the way home with a bursting stomach, two empty snack bags, and one disturbing mission.

The bathroom was pristine and spotless. I had recently bleached every inch of tile and porcelain. I made a promise not to contaminate my new bathroom. I vowed never to purge in there; this bathroom would remain pure, virtuous, and sinless.

To honor this vow, I ran downstairs and corrupted the half bathroom in the basement. This broke my bulimic seal. I drew pleasure and instant gratification from binging and purging. I rationalized that it was the lesser of my two evils. I convinced my diseased brain that purging reinforced my sobriety. It was my crutch and my distraction. Bulimia was my scapegoat.

It gave me the same anticipation as alcohol, yet it didn't destroy my life. The adrenaline rush was comparable and the high was identical. This didn't constitute a relapse. It was coping; it was my survival. It was always fucking *something*. Why couldn't I just be normal?

CHAPTER 17

Relapse Central Station

I sought sober support via social media. I felt a weight lifted from my shoulders when I made my first post proclaiming my sobriety. Admitting to the world that you're an alcoholic is the bravest and boldest footstep regarding initial sobriety. My Instagram was an illustration of my life. It was a portal, full of photos of myself drinking and having fun. Partying was my identity for five years. It defined who I was as a provocative and attractive young female.

I was the epitome of a party girl. Girls envied my flawless body, tanned skin, and golden locks. Men wanted to date me, and strangers wanted to converse with me. I was a head-turner and party-surfer. I was an attention whore with a genuine and hypersensitive core. Outwardly, I rendered superficial messages, but my intentions were deep and pure. This party girl façade was all a ruse. It was a distraction from my jagged reality. It was just a shell, protecting my heart and soul from any further damage.

I was a retracted turtle, hiding in my shell, protecting myself from predators. The more I played this fake and fictitious persona, the less vulnerable I felt as a woman. For years, I safeguarded and self-defended my fragile feelings. It was time to reveal to the world my raw and organic identity. This was my definition of sober—raw and organic. It's a person's feelings, thoughts, and emotions, unadulterated and not manipulated by a substance that changes those features. When you're drunk, your whole mind is not your own; it belongs partially to alcohol. And the more you drink, the more of your mind it possesses. For an alcoholic, this is devastating. We don't stop drinking. Therefore, our mind becomes a total slave to alcohol every time we drink.

Drugs and alcohol unequivocally alter your authentic personality, which varies from person to person. Alcohol afflicts everyone differently, and although it enhances some people, it is ultimately a depressant. It's the nature of the poison.

My very first sobriety post on Instagram read:

"Surrender to what is, let go of what was, have faith in what will be." #soberlife #sobersaturday #loveyourself #loveyourbody #lifestylechanges #mybodyismycanvas #fitandfab #soberissexy #movingforward #livingforme #goodbyeparty

This post exemplified my honest pursuit of sobriety. I would never post another picture of myself at a party or clutching a drink. My fresh, sober persona was undergoing inception. I felt a sense of liberation and redemption. I was enthusiastic, yet fearful for my future. I was treading in treacherous waters. I was exploring uncharted territory.

Exactly one month into my sober journey, I didn't just fall off the wagon; I tucked and rolled. It was a Friday and I had just gotten out of work. I was in high spirits because I had the weekend off. I set off on foot to the Italian deli down the street. As I passed the liquor store, I fantasized about drinking one, single airplane bottle. I stopped dead in my tracks. The plastic bags of Italian groceries I was carrying were heavy and flimsy. I gently placed them on the scorching, hot sidewalk as I readjusted my thoughts. The little devil on my right shoulder started babbling. The little guy convinced me that I could have one drink. My own brain was sabotaging me. It was undermining my sober endeavors; it didn't want me to succeed.

When I glanced back at the liquor store, my adrenaline started to pump. The *Open* sign was seducing me and flirtatiously whispering my name. The mere thought of being devious and sneaky aroused me. I was bored and I wanted to get away with something. My brain kept echoing the same mendacities: "You can have one drink. You deserve one drink." Addiction is literally the only disease that tries to convince you that you don't have it. I had a disease; I was in remission. My outlook was promising; I was happy and healthy.

Despite this progress, I chose to play the deadly game. I left the plastic bags filled with my groceries on the sidewalk, and I walked inside the liquor store. I had reached the point of no return. I was invested; I had to make the purchase. The musty, squalid smell of old cigarettes and cardboard boxes was classic. I had missed it. I was the only human on this planet who loved the smell of the liquor store. I don't know if it was a perceived association with alcohol or if I truly enjoyed the stale smell. Regardless, I was in heaven. I asked the attendant for two airplane bottles of coconut Cîroc and a pint of Smirnoff.

I shoved the goodies into my purse with pure exhilaration and a fire in my eyes. I swooped up the bags that were littering the sidewalk and started hiking home. My batteries were so charged, I couldn't wait any longer. I reached into my purse and felt around for the miniature, oblong bottle. The tiny bottle was so cute. I cracked it open and slammed it down the hatch before I had time to regret my decision.

I'm not sure why I had stepped foot into the liquor store that day. I was having a perfectly ordinary day. I wasn't depressed, distraught, or even angry. In fact, I was joyful. What goes on inside of an alcoholic's mind prior to relapse is incomprehensible and perplexing. The only word that I can utilize to clarify my rationale as an alcoholic is *mindfuck*. Your mind literally fucks with you and provokes you to use despite catastrophic consequences. My brain was uniquely wired. I didn't give a fuck about anything but the instant gratification. I wanted everything and I wanted it now. It is the disease of *more*.

I drank the entire weekend. It was Sunday and I couldn't fathom going back to work on Monday. When you're on a bender, long or short, the thought of resuming normalcy is implausible and unmanageable. The mere thought gave me tremendous anxiety. I got so engrossed into drinking that I lost touch with reality. For three days, I detached from my cognizance and numbed my thoughts and feelings. My ability to adhere back to realism was flawed. Normal people recoup from a weekend of partying and jump right back into their routine. I was abnormal. I was maladjusted.

I was walking home from Walgreens around eight on Sunday night. I was wearing my pink, fuzzy slides with spandex shorts that resembled underwear and a tight white spaghetti-strap with no bra. I was desperate for more alcohol because I had the Sunday blues. I abruptly left my house, pajamas and all; I was on a serious mission.

I purchased a six-pack of some craft beer, which was completely out of character for a seasoned junkie like myself. I wanted to enjoy a beer during my brief excursion home. When I tried to screw off the cap, it didn't budge. Perhaps I was too intoxicated, and my strength was curbed. When I realized I needed a bottle opener, I got angry. I started bashing the neck of the bottle, near the aperture, on the cement railing that was conveniently lining the sidewalk. After ten minutes, the bottle spurted open and beer flooded the sidewalk. I was too drunk for that shit. I pulled a 180 and returned to Walgreens. For round two, I purchased the cheapest bottle of white wine that featured a twist-off cap. I had just passed through the automatic sliding doors before I started chugging from the bottle. I stopped at the neighboring deli for God knows what. The night went black. The lights in my mind were flipped off. It was pitch dark.

I woke up around 7 a.m. in a bed at Flushing Hospital Medical Center. When I regained consciousness, my tantrum was initiated. I was affixed to a machine that was tracking my vitals, and an IV was fastened into my arm. Since I moved to New York, this was my eighth visit to the hospital, exclusively alcohol related. Seven of those hospital stints required a stretcher and an ambulance. I started squirming and wriggling out of the hospital bed. I literally expunged the IV out of my vein and ripped off the sticky electrodes that were adhered to my chest. I swiped my bag of clothes that were sitting next to the bed, hurriedly changed, and walked casually out of the building.

As I walked down the street, I kept looking back over my shoulder at the entrance to ensure that no clinical staff was pursuing me. This wasn't my first rodeo. Some hospitals follow a strict protocol for discharging patients, and I needed to be at work in three hours; I had no time to dillydally. I was on an impossible mission to make the 9:55 a.m. train to Penn Station. Luckily, I was still marginally drunk. This meant that my hangover was waiting in the wings. I knew it would emerge at the most inopportune hour. I brought a half bottle of Smirnoff to work to ensure a modest performance.

By the time my shift was over, I was moderately intoxicated. My pocket-sized, plastic bottle was empty, and I needed more. I ran across the street and scored a small bottle of Tito's. This bottle was glass and felt high-class. It certainly outclassed my usual plastic bum bottle. This was also enough vodka to last me for a whole day. I felt satisfied and reassured. On the train, I sipped from my bottle the entire way home. When I stood up to get off at my stop, I swayed back and forth. I was unsteady on my feet; even a gust of wind would have toppled me over. I walked down the steps of the station with precision and caution. The steps felt like an eternity. By the time I docked on the ground platform, I needed another drink.

My next move was something completely out of the ordinary. I walked into a bar and ordered a drink. Early in my drinking career, I exclusively drank at bars, clubs, and restaurants. I seldom consumed alcohol in my home, and if I did, it was with company. As a progressed alcoholic, I adopted a strict "no drinking in bars" policy. This ensured fewer hospital visits and less public humiliation. Granted, I was hospitalized nine times, but if it weren't for my policy, that number could have been closer to twenty.

I sat on a cruddy bar stool that showcased a ripped, maroon, upholstered seat. The seat itself was comfortable, but the legs were shaky and unstable. I couldn't figure out if the swaying back and forth was the chair or my drunk self.

Every patron in the bar was fixated on me. I was a fish out of water. They were all scruffy, middle-aged men who carried a few extra pounds. This hole-in-the-wall was their watering hole. I was a stray sunbird, casually slurping from their well. They weren't upset about it. Outwardly, we looked like different species of animals. I was a dainty bird and they were beasty hippos. We were *all* alcoholics. We were all peas in the same pod, cut from the same cloth, and had our hands in the same glove.

I blacked out approximately ten minutes after sitting my happy butt on that sketchy stool. Four hours later, I vaguely remember knocking on someone's door, thinking it was my house. The duplex looked identical to mine. It bore the same, light brick face, analogous stone railings, and matching window structures. Even the door looked similar. Throw a bottle of booze on top, and I thought this was my house. When I went to open the side door, it was locked. I huffed and puffed in aggravation as I swung around to the front door. It was also locked. I was even more aggravated.

I started banging on the screened door yelling, "Let me in." Two minutes later, a miniature Asian man opened the door without hesitation. I asked him why he was in my house. He politely responded, "This is my house." I was baffled. When I peeked inside, I noticed Asian trinkets and foreign artwork that overcrowded the walls. I also got jilted with a whiff of beef lo mein, egg drop soup, and soy sauce. This was clearly not my dwelling. The man was polite and even more confused than I was. He could tell that I was inebriated. He offered me help, which he later regretted.

I started sobbing profusely. I was crying like a toddler who had lost her mom in a grocery store. I was physically and mentally lost. I was disoriented, dejected, and deserted. I disrupted this poor man's peaceful evening.

We hopped into the man's 2000 Oldsmobile Silhouette minivan. It reeked of wontons and hot garbage, which I expected, considering the van's old age. I still had a Florida ID, so my attempt to remember my own address was futile. I was a mess.

We combed every block within a three-mile radius. He was driving the van, and I was driving him crazy. Every house that we passed I would perk up and holler, "That's it!" I then proceeded with, "Oh wait, never mind. That's not it." I repeated this nonsense for fifteen minutes until I noticed my roommates' charcoal-colored BMW stationed in the drive. "That's definitely it!" I shrieked. My tears dried up and I collected myself. I was praying that my roommate wasn't looking out the window. I wasn't a good liar when I was wasted, and I wasn't sure I could explain why an old Asian man was dropping me off. My roommate was usually passed out from smoking too much weed. I thanked the man profusely. I swung open the door and discreetly slithered inside. I heard the van's tires screeching away.

I continuously and unintentionally disrupted the lives of innocent and unsuspecting souls. During active addiction, I was careless and selfish. The world revolved around me and my life. I was used to people, primarily men, dropping everything and helping me. I was spoiled by the universe and I had no boundaries. My alcoholism brought out this egocentric, spoiled little brat. It brought out my juvenile side. I despised this girl, even more than I despised my sober self. I never wanted to be that girl. And, I would continue being that girl if I kept choosing to pick up the damn bottle.

CHAPTER 18

Blood, Sweat, and Rehab

Two days after my wild goose chase with the tiny Asian man, I returned to work. I was still on a bender because I couldn't stop. I was obliged to maintain my inebriation throughout my work shift. This was an art. One swig too many and I was passed-out drunk; one swig short and I was a trembling mess. On this day, I arrived equipped with the usual suspects, a pint of Smirnoff and a Vitamin Water. I was behaving sloppy as I heavyhanded my vodka into my Vitamin Water. I hadn't poured out enough of the water and the vodka spilled over. I chugged the rest of the alcohol that was in the pint. That was my first fatal error.

I was drunk and highly functional. The restaurant got slammed and I stepped up my game. I was dropping food off at tables and practicing my hospitality. The turn of events occurred immediately after I took a pickle-back shot with one of my tables. It punched me in the face, and

I was feeling groovy. My coworkers and I were nearing the end of our day shifts and our open tables were reduced to one. I was drunk and attempting to make my coworkers laugh. I was itching for a belly-aching laugh.

I started mocking the walk of a server who worked with us whom we were all friends with. This girl's name was Abigail. She was leggy and as thin as a rail. She was a square and also a goody-two-shoes. Her prude, uptight demeanor made her an ideal and professional waitress. She had a stick up her butt. My stick was in my hand. I was rebellious and sought laughter at other peoples' expense. I started pacing back and forth with a tray in my hand. I was mimicking Abigail's robotic saunter. Her back was always straight as a board and she resembled a Queen's Guard with a bearskin hat. She rendered an identical stoic and apathetic attitude. My coworkers were discreetly snickering with unmistakable grins on their faces. As this mockery was taking place, Abigail came marching up the stairs, like a British soldier.

She couldn't miss the laughter. She looked at me and knew precisely what was happening. She was a highly intelligent and perceptive girl. She stormed into the bathroom. My coworker, who must have sniffed my water bottle, interpreted my state. I was teetering back and forth between consciousness and comatose.

She gave me strict instructions. She called me an Uber and ordered me downstairs. She shoved me into the car and warned me not to pass go and collect $200. I was thoroughly advised to go straight home and sleep off whatever I had drunk. She would call me in an hour to ensure my safe arrival. I trusted her. I reluctantly climbed into the Hyundai Sonata. The Uber smelled like cigarettes and Lysol. I asked the driver to stop at Taco Bell, but he pretended like he didn't speak a lick of English. I leaned my head against the leather panel of the door and dozed off.

When I arrived home, I was completely oblivious to the calamity that I had just caused at my job. When I was drinking, I underestimated the pain that I inflicted on people. I lacked compassion and I lacked kindness. I was a monster, disguised in daisy dukes.

My Vitamin Zero bottle was empty and so was my heart. I needed more alcohol. I checked all my roommate's alcohol bottles. He had fancy bottles of Johnnie Walker Platinum, Grey Goose, and Patron that were displayed in the dining room. They were practically empty. Every time I would swig from one of his bottles, I would refill it with cheaper shit. Sometimes I even diluted the contents with water. Weeks later when I was desperate for alcohol I would swig from that same bottle and realize that it was mostly water. This would send me into a tailspin straight to the liquor store.

I checked the dishwasher and my closet. I often stashed bottles in bizarre and unsuspecting nooks and crannies. I hid the bottles from Avi because he knew that I was attempting the whole sobriety thing. I rustled around in my bedroom and struck gold. Underneath my bed was half a bottle of Tito's Vodka. I opened the brass-colored cap and sniffed it to confirm it was booze. I swigged the warm and mighty liquid. It was sweet and savory to my senses. I sat on my bearskin rug and processed the moment. I felt empty and alone.

When I woke up the following morning, I was in the hospital. There was a bright light staring me in the face. The doctor explained to me that I had fallen and busted my chin. He was about to stitch up my wound. He warned me that I would feel tugging and pulling. Ten minutes and five stitches later, I felt reassured that I could return home soon. I knew the drill. Three out of the nine hospital stints involved stitches and some sort of latent injury.

The only difference with this visit was that I was in a detox unit. Hours later, an Indian doctor visited me and tried to scare me with the classic "fatty liver speech" that I'd heard a thousand times before. He explained that my alcohol abuse was affecting my liver function. He blurted something out regarding the destruction of my liver cells, which results in scarring, and alcoholic hepatitis, which progresses from a fatty liver. I felt scared. I didn't want to die. I also felt angry because I didn't know how I'd landed in the hospital. I took an educated guess.

Allegedly, my roommate had arrived home from work around 10 p.m. He walked through the front door and was greeted by the smell of blood and Pizza Hut. I was lying perpendicular to the marble coffee table, drenched in blood. Our house looked like a crime scene. Bloody handprints marked up the white walls, and empty food wrappers littered the freshly mopped floor. My roommate had discovered my lifeless body and thought that someone had broken in and murdered me. He called 9-1-1 and the investigation launched. He told the cops that I was an alcoholic, and after a proper evaluation of the evidence, the scene was classified as an accident.

Back in the hospital, I was feeling progressively better. The nurse was nourishing my IV with saline and Benzodiazepines. The Benzos were administered to prevent acute alcohol withdrawal. These symptoms included delirium tremens, hallucinations, and tremors. It was over ten hours since I had my last drink and I was already entering a full-fledged withdrawal. This was the first time in my life that I didn't try to escape. I was in the right place; I knew I needed to detox.

I knew my roommate was pissed. I couldn't just stroll home and pretend like nothing had happened. I needed to face my consequences for once in my life. I also didn't want to clean up that mess; we needed a crime scene cleanup crew.

I remember lying on that hospital bed feeling like my mind was in a knot. I was seeing little thread-like strings hanging from the white ceiling panels. I was also convinced that the hospital was infested with bugs. I saw tiny ant-like critters scattering across the white walls. I was even hearing dull voices echoing in my ear. Despite the Valium, I was in full psychosis.

Every minute that passed felt like an hour. The cruel and agonizing day faded into a sleepless night. The stale hospital sheets were drenched in sweat. I was experiencing extreme temperatures, preceded by unbearable cold sweats. My body temperate was more unstable than a homeless crack addict's. My mood was swinging swifter than a wrecking ball, and my mind was spiraling faster than a hurricane. I was a mess and not a hot one.

My twin sister called me that evening. She understood the pain that I was in because she was also an alcoholic. She had just picked up her ninety-day chip and was on an optimistic road to recovery. She was living in a halfway house in south Florida and had just gotten a job at an animal shelter.

I heard her soothing voice and immediately started bawling. Having a twin sister was a unique experience. We had an undeniable connection; our souls were intertwined. Her voice was like a warm blanket that engrossed my broken body. I was so embarrassed that I had caused such a scene, literally a crime scene. She revealed that she had a surprise for me. She had secured a bed at a treatment center in Fort Lauderdale, Florida. It was the same treatment center that she had graduated from just two months prior. Apparently, Avi had called her to explain my desperate situation. She spoke to some people, pulled a few strings, and hooked me up. I didn't have health insurance and she reassured me that I would be receiving a scholarship, which translated to free rehab. My jaw hit the floor and I didn't even notice the threads hanging from the ceiling anymore. My response was a big, fat "Yes." I wept that entire night and fantasized about rehab.

My roommate came to swoop me up from the hospital to transport me directly to the airport. I hopped into his compact, two-seater Beamer and saw a packed bag beneath my feet. I knew it was mine. My roommate reinforced that we were not stopping at home under any circumstance. I didn't know if it was because he didn't want me drinking and/or running away or because the house still looked like a crime scene and he was protecting me. Either way, I conceded. It was the least I could do after the trauma that I had precipitated. On the way there, we smoked a blunt and hit the McDonald's drive-thru. I attacked a Big Mac and a large fries. I washed the grease down with an oversized Diet Coke.

When we arrived at the Departures gate, I slicked my blood-soaked hair back into a lime green scrunchy. I looked like the walking dead. I was too anxious and tense to notice the blood-stained shirt that I was sporting. I refused to shower in the hospital and was now paying the price. I said my goodbyes to Avi and my half-full Diet Coke. I promised him that I would return to New York a new woman. He was sympathetic and encouraging. He handed me a single, crisp hundred-dollar bill in case I got hungry. I think he just wanted me to get the fuck out of his car. He couldn't handle this degree of crazy.

I cleared security and beelined to the bar. I tried to purchase a whole bottle of vodka but realized it was only available as a checked item so I wouldn't be able to drink it until I landed in Florida. That would do me zero good. Instead, I sat at the bar and ordered a vodka soda. I sat there scrolling through Facebook and chugging my drink. I made this post on July 25, 2015:

I will be out of touch for a while. I've been trying to stay sober since March but my last slip just put me in the hospital covered in blood. I have an angel on my shoulder. This is so tough I can't even describe this feeling. I need to work a program so I can build a strong backbone. This substance destroys every aspect of who I am, including my appearance. I am unrecognizable. Bye for now, hello rehab.

Shortly after clicking the "post" button, I ordered two more drinks with the money I had left from the hundred. I got drunker faster than normal because of the barbiturates that were lingering in my system. I was not cognizant of my inebriation because when I went to board the plane, the attendant denied my entry. She called the paramedics claiming that I was "too intoxicated." I honestly don't remember being *that* drunk, but I also don't remember *everything*. The attendant sat me on a golf cart, and they wheeled me to a makeshift medical shack where they took my vitals. They immediately called the real paramedics because of my low blood pressure.

There I was, back in the same hospital, with the same nurses. I was more embarrassed than I was during the first go-around. I was forced to make the uncomfortable call to my roommate. He literally thought that I was playing an offensive and distasteful prank. I reiterated how serious I was and that he needed to rebook my flight because the airline refused to refund it based on the circumstances. He thought that he had gotten rid of me. Yet, I was back in his Beamer looking more rumpled than the night before.

He wasn't taking any chances. He purchased an airline ticket on the same flight as me. He held my hand as we walked though security to gate C23. I felt like a child, walking across a busy street holding my dad's hand. I was a dog on a leash. I was incompetent and sick. I was an alcoholic who desperately needed help.

CHAPTER 19

Riding in the Druggy Buggy

When I landed in Fort Lauderdale, I felt enthusiastic and eager, despite my grisly appearance and mediocre hygiene. I just had a few ruffled feathers and a stitched-up chin. Regardless, I was ready to tackle my addiction. I had no idea what to expect.

Crossing over from drunk to sober was easy. Acute withdrawal was physically painful, but it was time-sensitive. Having a finish line in sight made the process bearable. Sobriety, on the other hand, is a lifelong, daily endeavor. There was certainly no finish line. It wasn't solely about letting go of the bottle. It was more complicated and convoluted. The previous few months, I had been attempting to live dry. The struggle was real every single day that passed without alcohol.

There had to be an easier way to live. And that's exactly why I was so eager to come to rehab. I needed help because my way wasn't working. I was here to figure out the paradigm of sobriety and happiness.

The way that I was living was unmanageable regardless of whether I was sober or not. That didn't align with my rationale. How was my life still out of control even while I was sober? It sounded like a contradiction.

I quickly solved this confusion. Sobriety is the act of not drinking. I expected to stop drinking and live happily. Recovery is characterized by what an individual does with their life as a sober entity. That's exactly why I came to treatment. I needed to explore the tools of my individual recovery. Sobriety is simply a tool of recovery.

My life wasn't working for me. I had a job, an apartment, and a life, but I wasn't fulfilled. Most addicts must lose everything before they choose to get help. From the outside, I hadn't lost everything. Internally, I had lost myself, which meant everything. I had lost my compassion, my selflessness, my loyalty, and my genuine smile. Losing those virtues *were* my rock bottom. I was a diamond with no luster.

I walked through the doors of East Coast Recovery on July 20th and my whole soul was lost. I didn't know where I was going in life and I didn't know who I was as a woman. Chasing things that I presumed would make me happy had been my downfall. This chase exhausted me. It broke me.

Up until this point, my life was a relentless chase. I chased fifteen minutes of fame, hoping that notoriety would fulfill me. I chased New York, expecting to live a happy life. I chased men and I chased men with money. I thought that if I could just have Brooks, I would be happy. I chased alcohol and food, which I used to cope. I kept chasing these illusions; I was like a dog chasing my own tail. There was nothing to catch. I toyed with the notion of accepting happiness, in that moment, regardless of where I was at in life. This notion adhered to my brain and I thought about it every day.

The first thing I did when I arrived at the rehab was count my blessings, because I had been given many chances and I was certainly grateful to be alive.

I was called into a room with nothing on the wall except a poster that read, "It's a beautiful day to be sober." That sign irritated me. It was a flat-out lie. Just because I was sober didn't mean my day was beautiful. I could recall a hundred sober days that were ugly. When I was finished overanalyzing an innocent, motivational poster, I was required to take an assessment, which consisted of a thousand personal questions regarding my addiction. Even though the assessment was a sequence of questions, it was pushy and aggressive. It was violating my addiction. My alcoholism wanted to be left in a corner and it wanted to be isolated. And now, it was being addressed. All eyes were on my addiction. It was in the hot seat and I was forced to answer all the tough questions.

When the initial intake was completed, I felt a weight lifted off my shoulders as well as some persistent withdrawal symptoms. My palms were clammy, and my forehead was sweaty. I wasn't sure if it was the angst from the new environment or the withdrawal. Regardless, I was feeling shitty. My mood was volatile and unpredictable. A fellow patient asked me how I got the stitches on my chin and I responded, "Take a guess." He replied, "Um, I don't know." Then I said, "I'm a freaking alcoholic and I'm in rehab. I obviously fell." Then he had the nerve to ask me, "How?" I gave him the cold shoulder and stomped away like a child having a tantrum. I needed to be alone before I made any more enemies.

Next, it was time for me to go back to the all-female house where I would be staying. I jumped in a giant white cargo van, also known as the "druggy buggy." The proper definition of a druggy buggy was a vehicle that transported drug addicts.

When the buggy pulled up to the house, I was pleasantly surprised. Probably because I was accustomed to living in a shoebox in New York City. This was not a shoebox; this was an actual house, with windows and a roof. The house itself was charming and practical. It featured a sizable open kitchen with an island and two spacious living rooms with sixty-inch flat screens. We had every available channel known to man. The only caveat was the parental controls. Apparently, we were categorized as children. I appreciated this assumption. We were a flock of drug addicts; we were emotionally and mentally stifled.

The first thing I did was jump into the shower. My hair was caked with crusty, dried blood. I will never forget the putrid smell of rotten blood as I stood under the showerhead. It made me want to vomit, even today. I remember watching the water beneath my feet turn orange. As disturbing as this was, I felt empowered. That smell reassured me that I was in the right place—under the shower, cleansing my evils. Watching the reddish, orange water draw into the tiny, rusted drain was cathartic. I was witnessing my past slowly wash away. The wounds from my alcoholism had bled for many years; that blood was now saturating my shower. All my pain, hatred, anger, and sadness that my addiction spawned was being flushed down the drain. When I stepped onto the filthy bathroom mat, I felt like a new woman. I felt invigorated and energized. I felt clean and I was ready to heal the wounds.

There were approximately twelve other females in the program, ranging in age from eighteen to sixty. There were two categories: the alcoholics and the drug addicts. The drug addicts were hardcore. I had never met a person who shot heroin. These girls were younger than me with track marks lining the inside of their arms. The newcomers, like myself, were sickly looking. They looked like they hadn't eaten for months. My reason for being so thin wasn't because of drugs. I was the only one who suffered from an eating disorder. I felt special.

The fellow alcoholics of the group were interesting characters. There was a hilarious African American lady whom we called Aunt Jemimah. She was a fifty-year-old Walgreens employee. Her specialty was in the beauty department. She brought a suitcase full of Moroccan oil, shampoo, and conditioner for "women of color," and cocoa butter lotion. She smelled like a walking coconut. She had been drinking a gallon of vodka a day for seven years and still managed to hold down a job. She was impressive in every way. She braided everyone's hair and cooked us her famous southern staples including fried chicken, green bean casserole, and homemade grits.

The other alcoholic was around the same age. He owned a trailer in Indiana and proudly displayed the American flag on every piece of clothing he wore. He had drunk a case of Budweiser every night and was court-ordered to rehab after accumulating four DUIs. Every day, he complained about his tax situation. Apparently, he owed thousands to the IRS and his paychecks were being garnished. I felt bad for the guy, but we all had our own unique problems. His just sucked a little worse.

Four of the female heroin addicts were best friends. They were immature nineteen-years-olds who had been in and out of rehab. They knew the ins and outs and plotted against the staff. Their conversations consisted of boys, makeup, and clothes. They were all super-skinny when they were using heroin and had gained at least twenty-five pounds since they got clean. Regardless, they squeezed into their old jeans and small tanks. They disregarded the dress code and flaunted their muffin tops and flabby stomachs. My attempts to hang with them quickly ceased when I overhead a conversation they were having about giving each other matching tattoos by using a needle and pen ink. I wasn't going to get suckered into a botched tattoo or a shoddy piercing. Hell to the no.

There were only a few patients I had anything in common with. A girl named Ashley shared the same sense of humor. She was intelligent, motivated, and outgoing. She was successful and beautiful. She had gotten in a car accident and was prescribed Tramadol. She continued the medication even after the pain had subsided. Her incredibly high tolerance had compelled her to start snorting the pills. She used narcotics for two years before her husband gave her an ultimatum. It was either treatment or divorce. I was happy that she chose rehab. She was my saving grace.

The treatment center spoiled us like little children. Every move we made was being monitored. We were always accompanied by a technician to ensure appropriate conduct and acceptable behavior. Every week, the technicians drove us to Publix, where we were given $100 for grocery shopping. Certain items were restricted like candy and Advil. They also drove us to the gym every day. I never went because we were only allowed to go for twenty minutes. That amount of time was futile. Weekends were predominantly non-clinical—no therapy on Saturday and Sunday. Saturday was an outing day; i.e., fishing, bowling, sailing, etc. The field trips, the constant chaperoning, the recess smoke breaks, and the regulated snacking made me feel like a child in elementary school. The only element we were missing was naptime.

I was thriving in the treatment environment. I was participating in groups, journaling extensively, and expressing my multitude of emotions. One minute I was sobbing hysterically; two minutes later I was laughing uncontrollably. I sorted through an incredible spectrum of emotions. I poked into my past and I dug into my soul. It was just the inception of my soul searching. I addressed my childhood trauma and tackled my intrusive thoughts. This was just grazing the surface. Staying sober in a regulated, controlled environment was the easy part. Staying sober in a world laced with triggers and traps would prove daunting.

One week into treatment, I was called to the office. The staff proceeded to explicate how well I was progressing in the program. They said I was ready to step down into sober living. I experienced two emotions in the moment, enthusiasm and disappointment. I was the *one* person who didn't want to escape from the center, yet I was being forcefully discharged. I wanted to stay for thirty days. Maximizing my time and optimizing my stay was a priority. And now, I was being thrown out to the curb with my suitcase and a bus pass. I was an exemplar student. I was cooperative and diligent and I was also a scholarship. Therefore, I was not paying a dime. The beds were all full and they needed room for the incoming clients. They cleaned house and replaced me with an individual with a fat insurance policy. I was slightly hurt and offended, yet, grateful for those seven days. I always wonder, what if I had stayed the entire thirty days? Perhaps I wouldn't have relapsed less than a year later.

CHAPTER 20

Sober-Livin' the Life

I had been left in the dust. I wheeled my busted suitcase into the halfway house where I would be living for, hopefully longer than a week. I was now a paying customer, which offered me security. I was attending AA meetings every day and I felt sturdy in my sobriety. Staying sober in an environment that held me accountable proved vital. I needed this liability and supervision. My selfishness and stealth didn't disappear overnight. I was on the pink cloud of treatment. I was walking the walk and talking the talk. I was confident, yet arrogant. I thought I had this recovery thing in the bag. Two weeks out and I felt like a walking success story, but I wasn't winning. I was making loser decisions. Decisions that certainly didn't align with recovery and didn't align with the twelve-step program.

Instead of swallowing my pride and seeking a low-key job at a restaurant, I dated older men for money. I refused to work. I wanted to have my cake and eat it too. I was a cheater, just like Brooks. Although I was sober, I was still addicted. I was addicted to the thrill of these men and the money they threw at me. I was one drink away from working as a stripper. I progressively stopped attending meetings and started running upwards of ten miles daily. I was thin and I had money in the bank. I was disillusioned and jaded. This felt like success but I had regressed.

I was consistently lying to my friends, my family, and my house mom. Most importantly, I was lying to myself. The more I lied, the sicker I became. I was binging and purging every other day and I felt broken. I needed to push the "restart" button. Because I was sober, I was cognizant of what was happening. I reeled myself back into recovery.

Two months after my discharge from rehab, I accepted a job at Texas De Brazil. I used my last $600 from a sugar daddy and purchased a scooter. I was busting my butt and attending AA meetings. I was back on track, but I wrestled daily with my eating disorder. Working at Texas De Brazil proved challenging for a veteran bulimic.

At the end of the night, we were given every ounce of leftover food. We feasted and devoured all this delicious food, every night. For a bulimic, this was poison. A normal person knows when to stop eating. A bulimic's brain never turns that button off. My brain told me to keep eating until I couldn't breathe. It anticipated a purge because that's what it was trained to do.

There were many nights I forced myself to slither out of the restaurant before the temptation arose. Then there were other nights when I gorged on cheese bread, mashed potatoes, steak, chicken, lamb chops, soups, and fancy cheeses. Then I hustled dangerously home on my scooter, swerving in and out of traffic, with no helmet. When I got back, I turned the shower and the sink faucet on simultaneously while I did the disgusting deed. Immediately after, I felt satisfied and dissatisfied synchronously. I was relieved that it was over, yet angry at myself for exhibiting self-destructive behavior. I promised myself that I would never purge again; It was physically painful and mentally malicious.

Four months after I started legitimately and laboriously working, I met a man whom I really liked named Mark. He was an older guy who had his shit together. He lived in a luxurious, posh condo on Fort Lauderdale Beach. He was a divorcee with two grown children. On paper, Mark checked off all the boxes. He was respectful, charming, successful, and generous. I wondered why he was single; within a few weeks that answer was crystal clear.

I couldn't be honest with Mark regarding my past. I circumnavigated the truth regarding my sobriety. Our first genuine conversation occurred while dining at the Seasons 52 restaurant. I ordered a flatbread and a Diet Coke. He found it refreshing that I refused an alcoholic beverage. I stuck my toe in the water regarding the sobriety conversation, simply to gauge his reaction. I expressed that my twin sister was sober and in a halfway house. This was a true statement. I neglected to mention that I was also riding on that same wagon. The word "halfway house" freaked him out; I could see the judgment in his eyes. He probably pictured a rundown shack in a low-income neighborhood infested with drug addicts. I read his movements and evaluated his responses.

I reminded myself that he was twice my age. He didn't comprehend addiction especially in this generation. His life was relatively idyllic. He had a fairly normal family with over-achieving children who were my age. Unless you've been exposed directly to addiction, you don't truly grasp the nature of the disease. I could tell that he affiliated addiction and sobriety with the stereotypes that society has generously produced. I didn't fault him. This was not even the straw that broke the camel's back.

The way that Mark spoke to me was off-putting. He was one of those old-fashioned men who expected me to be at his beck and call, 24/7. Keep in mind, this was impossible while living in sober living. There were rules to follow and conduct to uphold. There were curfews and regulations. Dating was highly frowned upon during the first year of recovery. This was the number two rule that I was breaking from day one. The number one rule was obvious—no using drugs or alcohol.

One day, I hopped on my scooter and headed to Mark's condo. My scooter broke down, right in the middle of a high-traffic street. In South Florida, every street was congested. I pushed the sucker to the median and placed a call to Mark, informing him of my mishap. His response was,

"So do you think you're going to make it or not?" Then, he proceeded to reproach me. He rambled on about how this was the second time we had made plans that had fallen through. My scooter was fucking smoking on the side of the road and this man was irate that we weren't hanging out?! I couldn't make this stuff up.

It was an accumulation of minor events that led me to end our not-so-whirlwind romance. The only perk of the relationship was his brand-new Porsche convertible that I couldn't even drive. I preferred the wind in my hair on my own scooter. The car, the condo, and the gifts weren't worth the hassle that this man created.

Aside from his annoying attitude, it was another man that compelled me to cut ties. My new man was in recovery, just like me. This guy, Stefan, didn't have all the bells and whistles, but he was genuine, humble, and compassionate. He wasn't financially stable, but he was emotionally stable. He was generous with what few dollars he had. What he did offer was emotional support, empathy, kindness, and a unique optimism. Those qualities meant more to me than wads of cash. He was just special.

I was upfront and honest. I explained to Mark that I had met a man whom I had a stronger connection with. He was appalled and outraged. He couldn't fathom that I had found someone *better* than him. He reminded me that he was the whole package. I didn't want his package. It was crap.

Mark reacted to this news like a bitter teenaged boy. He made comments like, "Good luck with your drug addict boyfriend." And, "You're going to end up drinking soon anyways." He even requested that I return the gifts that he had purchased for me, including a Pandora bracelet and a Michael Kors watch. This junk probably totaled $200. Seriously?! This was a classic egomaniac who was not familiar with rejection. This solidified my decision. I gave the MK watch to my friend and lost the Pandora bracelet about two months later. Oh well.

Stefan was different. He was patient, polite, and understanding. He had battled his own addiction to pain pills and could relate to my alcoholism. I disclosed everything to this man. He listened with an open ear and an open heart. He wasn't egotistical and he certainly wasn't a pig. He spoke highly of women and never degraded them. He never even looked at another woman. He was respectful and respectable. He was a hidden gem among the recovery community. He was a diamond in the rough among society as a whole. He was bashful and nervous. This was a stark cry from the other arrogant and boisterous addicts who stuffed the rooms of AA and NA. And he wasn't sailing under false colors; he turned out to be the same exact person that he portrayed on day one.

CHAPTER 21

The Secret Letter

A few months into sobriety I was getting these awful visions from my past. I couldn't let go of the mistakes that I had made. I had ruined the lives of strangers and had broken every rule in the book. I was fixated on my faults. I had this robust urge to make things right. I wanted to apologize to every single person I had harmed. My sense of remorse was overpowering, and debilitating. I ended up writing the following letter to Brooks' wife to clear my conscience. It forced me to process the devastation that I had caused. This letter never left my computer screen, but it was proof of my intentions.

Dear Anne,

I know that it may seem unusual for me to write this letter 5 years after the affair but it's something I need to do for myself and hopefully will give you more closure. I'm working on my 9th Step in *Alcoholics Anonymous which involves making our amends to people we have hurt. As strange as it sounds, I want to apologize to you. Since, I got sober my guilt and shame has eaten me away. I literally think about my actions every single day. Whether you read this letter or not is your discretion, but I need to express my deepest shame.*

I moved to New York City in the winter of 2012 and met Brooks months later. I had $100 to my name and was desperate to make ends meet. When I met him, I was a child. I had just graduated from college and knew nothing about life and consequences. I had no respect for myself or anyone else for that matter. Brooks filled a void. As sick as it sounds, he was my father figure. A figure that has been absent for the past 5 years. He gave me money and attention which I frantically sought. I was obsessed with his money and addicted to attention and alcohol. I am an alcoholic and during that time, I was very sick in my disease. I had zero regard for other human beings. I had no friends or family in New York. My loneliness manifested into horrible choices. As you know, Brooks is a sick man. His own addiction to sex and alcohol made us two peas in a pod. I wanted everything that you had. I wanted the lifestyle that he provided. I thought that if I had everything that you had, I would be complete, and my life would be a dream.

As our relationship progressed, I became more and more reliant on Brooks and his money. I couldn't imagine getting through a week without his financial support. I went from having nothing to having everything. Or at least, I thought I had everything.

I threw away all of my morals, to become a materialistic, unemotional, cold person. Brooks convinced me we were soulmates and I, being freshly 24, believed every word that he said. To this day, I look back and recognize how his own alcoholism affected every aspect of his life. I clearly see now that he isn't this self-made, intelligent, family-oriented, funny and perfect man that I painted him as. He was sick and suffering. He was addicted to sex, money and alcohol. He was suffering from the same disease that I have been battling for over six years.

Alcoholism is a disease of more. We always want more even if we have everything in the world. Whether its caffeine, alcohol, sex or food, we are constantly seeking more, never truly satisfied until the next fix. It's a compulsion and obsession that normal people like yourself will never truly understand.

Brooks changed who I was as a person. His impact on my life was detrimental. He caused me immense pain even though your scars run deeper. Brooks made me believe that every man was perverted. He made me believe that having sex with him would give me everything in the world. All I had to do was sacrifice. I thought that I deserved to be treated with utter disrespect for myself and my body. I believed that the only thing I was good for was sex. He used me for this reason.

After getting sober, I realize that there are loyal men out there. I know I'm more than an object, I'm a human being who was fooled. My actions were absolutely disgusting. I am so sorry for being the woman that caused you so much pain. Women are supposed to stick together against the men that disrespect us, and what I did was a disgrace to femininity. I not only cheated myself, but I disappointed womankind.

Brooks' obsession with sex overrode his morals, loyalty and respect. His actions were destructive, and he knew the one thing that could rectify his errors was to avoid me, and he failed *miserably. I truly feel that his addiction was the reason for that. It affects the brain in numerous ways and makes us powerless over things that we crave. He was a very sick man and I pray from him to this day.*

He is a deeply hurt, sad and insecure man whose money and family are his only reasons for living. I believe that he loves you to death, but this disease makes you do things that are almost out of our control. I know that I spiraled out of control and so did my alcoholism. I deeply apologize for making you feel the way that you did. You are an incredible human who doesn't deserve to be treated the way that you were. I want to make an amends because that is what you deserve.

Through this disaster, I learned that money cannot buy happiness. The keys to happiness are loyalty, respect, love and sincerity. I regret the affair because I hurt someone who doesn't deserve pain. I just want you to know that it wasn't your fault, my fault or anyone else's fault for that matter. Brooks' behaviors and actions were solely his to choose and I'm embarrassed and ashamed that I participated in that. I pray for you and your family and wish true happiness within your heart.

-Brittany

CHAPTER 22

Love After Addiction

Finding love in the aftermath of addiction is like learning how to walk after losing both of your legs. You lose yourself in addiction. In recovery you explore the self-love, faith, and passion for life that your addiction took away. Then, you must transform those qualities into a love language that the other person understands via communication, emotional expression, and intimacy.

I was in a dysfunctional relationship with alcohol for five years. It controlled my every move. I became comfortable with submission and accepted the anguish. My self-love and self-worth faded along with my voice. Happiness was artificially derived due to the lack of human connection. My communication capabilities were curbed and my overall desire for relationships outside of the bottle was nonexistent. It was a lonely and empty relationship. Yet, I continued to choose the alcohol.

The bottle was a safe relationship for a girl fearful of rejection. It never criticized me. The bottle was reliable; it never left my side. And, when it did run low, I got more. It was replaceable. I had the power; I controlled where I drank, when I drank, and how much I drank. I controlled the physical bottle while the toxic contents controlled me.

How does an addict recover from this maladjustment? I grappled with this reality, as well as the reality of allowing another human into my life. I resisted strong and hard. I refused to let Stefan in. I was a castle surrounded by fortress walls, barbed wire, and a moat. Getting anywhere near my castle was half the battle. I fired cannons and Stefan still crawled closer. Fortunately, he was wearing heavy armor, because he survived my shots.

For five years, it was *my* life. I controlled every aspect as a selfish rebel. Now, I was expected to share my life? He didn't earn his way in. He just waltzed in like a ballroom dancer. I still wanted to live my way. Unfortunately, my way sucked, so I gave the poor guy a chance. And, as much as I didn't trust men, I sort of, kind of, trusted Stefan.

I clearly wasn't prepared to love because I didn't understand mutual feelings. I believed that nothing was ever mutual. I've always witnessed love accompanied by pain—it was present in every love story, even fairy tales. And remember, I avoided pain at any cost, even if it meant drowning myself out with alcohol. Sacrificing wasn't in my repertoire. The intended result of love wasn't worth any amount of pain.

Even though I avoided pain, my addiction left me with a high threshold and tolerance. For years, I practiced stonewalling and resistance. I bottled every emotion and swept all dirt under the rug; nothing was ever vacuumed. I pretended like nothing hurt even when I was completely broken. Stefan painlessly showed me how to love.

My past experiences with men were spins of the roulette wheel and the ball never landed on my color or number. I was utterly convinced that they were always the problem. I was *never* the common denominator. Men were the root of all evil. They were all sex-addicted, liars, and cheaters; Brooks was my proof. Then, Stefan rolls in and blasts my theory wide open. He was none of these things. Perhaps my thesis was defective. I needed more research.

When you get sober, you don't automatically become a good person. I know plenty of awful, sober people. Sobriety offers no guarantees regarding integrity. What does sobriety do? It gives you an opportunity and a fighting chance to become your best self. When you are using, personal growth is stunted. It's like being held back in the fourth grade, over and over again. When I got sober, I felt like I was in the fourth grade; I had so much work to do. I was playing catch-up. Stefan was my tutor. He challenged and pushed me.

Throughout my addiction, self-hatred was a prominent theme. Sobriety taught me how to *like* myself. During early sobriety, I *thought* I loved myself. Looking back now, I clearly didn't love myself because I continued to use my eating disorder as a coping mechanism. Stefan truly helped me love myself by allowing me to see what he saw, through his eyes. When I fell in love with myself, my eating disorder magically went quiet. It went from a loud rumble to a quiet purr. I still hear it, but I have learned to ignore it and it certainly doesn't dominate my life.

When I started dating Stefan, I had many uncertainties. I knew in my heart that I couldn't give him my soul because I was still soul searching. He was a good man, with a good heart. He was also loyal and trustworthy. I knew that I had work to do before I could start dating him. Regardless, I couldn't let him walk away and start dating another girl. I was selfish and refused to let him go. I liked myself enough to realize that I deserved him. I had faith and he had patience. Together, we worked.

Stefan was almost two years into his recovery, and I was just two months. This was an enormous discrepancy. He was mature, rational, and sturdy. I was not. Regardless, he precisely comprehended where I stood in my recovery. We were honest with each other about our broken pasts. He remained eager in his pursuit despite what he knew he was facing. I worshiped his maturity, wisdom, and perseverance and eventually learned to practice those abilities myself.

When Stefan met me, I was a promising little sprouted seed. I didn't know how to become a flower and I didn't allow anyone to water me. I waited. I realized I needed watering or I would never grow. I finally allowed Stefan to nourish me. He took delicate care. He watered me with compassion and provided me with optimism and sunlight.

I was a stubborn flower and required extra care. Two years later, and with a heavy dose of TLC, I grew into a beautiful flower. I trusted Stefan to nurture and protect my delicate little petals and he never even left the garden. Love is patient and kind. I am grateful.

CHAPTER 23

Alcoholism in an Alcoholic Society

Saying "goodbye" to alcohol was easy, but abstaining from alcohol was *not* easy. I comprehended the reality that I couldn't drink, but it was more complicated than that. I'm a thirty-year-old female in a society that glorifies drinking. Alcohol is socially acceptable despite its deadly reputation. It is normalized and mainstreamed. With this acceptance, we ignore the harm. I hear people say all the time, "It's just alcohol." True, it is *just* alcohol, but it also "just kills" a hundred thousand people each year.

Alcohol is literally everywhere, and Americans turn every occasion into a drinking occasion. I've seen alcohol at graduation parties, baby showers, children's parties, baptisms, and so on. I grew up in this standardized age of alcohol. It wasn't even a question of whether I was going to drink or not. I knew that if it was a gathering, there would be alcohol and I would be drinking. It honestly wasn't even a choice. It was more of an assumption. In college, my friends and I would drink every time a group of us got together; two was always a party. We drank at the movie theaters, at the beach, at the bowling alley, out to lunch, and even in the park playing frisbee. At what point does casual drinking turn into alcoholism?

Everyone denies that their drinking is problematic, simply because it's socially acceptable. Just for sake of argument, let's assume heroin became legal; Americans started shooting up during every occasion and it was normalized. It would not be problematic, right? Simply because something is socially accepted doesn't make it acceptable.

Let's look at social media. It is a parade of Americans abusing alcohol. There are girls sipping champagne by the pool and guys chugging beer during the game. This media appears frivolous and harmless. It's not the activity that is alarming; it's the frequency. Instagram is an infinite collection of photos and videos of people drinking. It's constant and never-ending. Drinking is a dominant commonality among many users. With hashtags like #winedown, #tequillatuesday, #wineoclock, and #margaritamonday, our generation is finding any and every opportunity to consume alcohol.

I hear people say all the time, "I don't need to drink." If you don't *need* to drink, then why did you choose to drink? Just because your body isn't physically dependent on alcohol doesn't mean you don't mentally need it to have a good time. Many people are under the assumption that if they don't drink every night, they're not alcoholics. This may be true, and this may not be true. Without a proper diagnosis, we can only speculate. Regardless, people need to realize that alcoholism isn't black or white.

We like to categorize drinkers into two categories, non-alcoholics and alcoholics. Binge drinkers rationalize how they don't fit into the alcoholic group simply because they don't drink every night. Therefore, they don't have a problem. What people fail to recognize is a vast, unexplored gray area of alcohol abuse. There is binge drinking, alcohol abuse, and alcohol dependence, which is your classic alcoholic. Some drinkers may fit into none of these categories, while some fit into all three.

We need to stop stigmatizing the word *alcoholic*. People hear that word and cringe. They get all defensive, just like I did during my drinking career. That word is fucking scary. No one wants to be labeled an alcoholic. That was a term used for old war veterans who sat in their rocking chair and drank whiskey all day. The reality is, we are a generation full of alcohol abusers.

No matter how flat you make a pancake, there's always two sides. Social media reinforces drinking, but it also supports sobriety. It allows us to connect with others who have similar struggles. It is also an infinite resource for knowledge associated with addiction. Since I got sober, Instagram has been my creed. The sober support that I receive is phenomenal. It's a therapeutic outlet for creative expression. I'm a relatively shy person. It's challenging for me to walk up and start a conversation with a total stranger. Social media enables me to reach out to people whom I normally wouldn't have connected with.

Society bears such a negative stigma on the interpretation of the word *alcoholic*. The word connotes secrecy, shame, and associated stereotypes. Paradoxically, the word *denotes* addiction and dependence. I am an alcoholic. I don't hide that fragment of my identity. I don't allow myself to feel shameful of my disease. My discreditable actions were a direct, merciless result of my sickness, which was instilled in my brain long before I picked up my first drink. Society has a disconnect regarding addiction as a psychological disease and the degrading stigma associated with the person afflicted, which is truly devastating to humanity. How are we able to admit to our problem and become sober if society stigmatizes us? Why not promote acceptance and awareness, which would allow us to become not only cognizant of our relationship with alcohol but proactive in recovery? Owning my addiction has manifested into this beautiful life of sobriety that I live today.

CHAPTER 24

Goodbye, Love

Sobriety challenges me every day. It is a part of my identity. Sobriety is a form of self-love. It forces you to look at yourself in the mirror without a filter. Sobriety represents simplicity. It's a natural form of myself, without the alteration of a substance. I'm forced to feel every raw emotion and deal with discomfort, awkwardness, and even sadness. Being in this state of mind allows me to build substantial and genuine connections with myself and other humans. Being yourself one hundred percent of the time is not easy, but it's worth it. Alcohol was my first love and that love is dead. All the energy that I utilized on alcohol can now be recycled. This twisted love story has a fairy tale ending. I wanted to end this story with a goodbye letter that I wrote in rehab. Alcohol may have been my first love, but I refused to make it my last.

Dear Alcohol,

You are everywhere. You leave your mark on everything. You are featured in lyrics, on billboards, on television and in magazines. You grace the shelves of every store and refrigerator. Your roar is impossible to ignore. Your exposure is high, but your potency and peril are severe. You're unpredictable, risky and fatal. You're the venom of a snake and I was blindly bitten. You casually slithered your way into my life. In fact, you slithered your way into every American household like an essential. You're a staple at every party and get-together. You know precisely how to initiate a party, but my party is over.

You were like candy to me. I couldn't have just one. You gave me confidence, washed away my worries and freed my fears. You were an illusion. In reality, you lowered my inhibitions, eradicated my expectations and transformed my clean conscience into a girl I don't even recognize. The false feelings and emotions you provided were a fantasy that manifested into a true nightmare. It was time to wake up.

Life without you is heaven on earth, most days. With you, I'm the devil, in hell. You will no longer demonize me. The ghosts you instigated will no longer haunt me. You are dead to me.

You left me for dead. You left me with physical and mental scars that can start healing. Every drop of blood and every tear I shed was not in vain. I learned who you were. Your temporary comfort and instant gratification were a sham. The scars on my body will remind me every day how destructive and malicious you truly are.

You possessed me for nearly five years, but I regained my consciousness. I reclaimed my power and will. I surrendered to my higher power, but I did not surrender to you. I will continue to fight and defeat you every single day, for the rest of my life.

You imprisoned me for five years. I regained control and arrested you. You deserve a life sentence. In fact, you deserve death. I'm executing you. It's you or me on death row and I choose you.

This eradication is permanent; this is your end and my beginning. Your death will give me life. A life of gratitude, bliss and most importantly, love. My future is bright because of the darkness that you cast on my life for too long. I refuse to live in your shadow. I am alive again. I am free.

About the Author

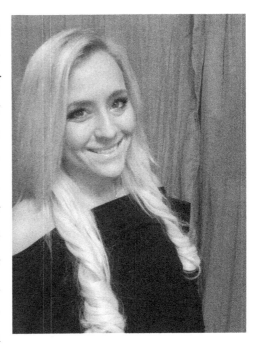

Brittany Taltos is an advocate for breaking the stigma of addiction. She uses her blog and social media to generate dialogue surrounding mental illness. She speaks candidly about her struggles to help others overcome their own challenges. Her enthusiasm, compassion, and optimism characterize her life in sobriety.

Prior to her recovery, Brittany was a bona fide party girl. During her early twenties, she and her twin sister, Erica, coined the term "Twinning" after appearing on Season 3 of *Jersey Shore*. She bombed another reality show, *Bachelor Pad*, becoming the most forgettable contestant. After managing to graduate from the University of Florida, she moved to New York City.

Armed with a degree in advertising, Brittany launched her alcoholic career by becoming a bartender. Within two years, she became a top blackout artist. She achieved eight alcohol-related hospital stints in four years and became a master of binge drinking. In 2016, she retired from drinking and moved to South Florida, where she sought treatment for her addiction.

In 2018, Brittany moved to New Jersey with her boyfriend. She currently works as an ophthalmic technician at a doctor's office. She loves her job and cannot imagine life without her Goldendoodle, her boyfriend, and her sobriety.

Find the Author

Website
https://girlwasted.com/

Instagram
https://www.instagram.com/sober_barbie_/

Facebook
https://www.facebook.com/brittany.leilanii

LinkedIn
www.linkedin.com/in/brittany-taltos-28026b45

Made in the USA
Las Vegas, NV
19 February 2024